DIET TO DETOX

DR ESE STACEY

DIET TO DETOX

DR ESE STACEY

To my children Luke, Harry and Hannah

Published in 2022 by SilverWood Books

SilverWood Books Ltd
14 Small Street, Bristol, BS1 1DE, United Kingdom
www.silverwoodbooks.co.uk

ISBN 978-1-80042-200-1 (paperback)
ISBN 978-1-80042-201-8 (ebook)

British Library Cataloguing in Publication Data
A CIP catalogue record for this book is
available from the British Library

Page design and typesetting by SilverWood Books

SilverWood

A NOTE FROM DR ESE

I qualified as a medical doctor in 1990. I trained at St. Mary's Hospital Medical School in London. St. Mary's Hospital Medical School was where Sir Alexander Fleming discovered penicillin. Little did I know that when we took classes in the famous lecture theatre named after him, I would be one day writing a book about gut microbes and the toxins that affect them.

It was my long-held dream to train to be a doctor who specialized in sport. I love sport and would dream of being a doctor to elite athletes. I am grateful that I was able to fulfil that dream. However, along the way, my three children came along. All with their specific health challenges, of which you will hear plenty whilst you read the book. My children's health problems began to open my mind to the fact that I hadn't been taught everything I needed to know about health. There I was, a consultant in the field of high performance sport and yet I was struggling to know what to do to help my children to function in day-to-day life. I'm grateful for this journey because not only has it allowed me to help my children to be well but it has allowed me to help you, the reader. The journey allowed me to see the crucial role played by the gut for general health. You'll read about this journey and what I learned along the way. The journey helped me to see that just about all sickness is related to the function of the gut and its microbes and toxins. In March 2019 in a moment of understanding, I was able to put all my ideas into a coherent picture which I call the Hierarchy of Health. Understanding the Hierarchy of Health enables you to skip huge chunks of medical knowledge. The Hierarchy of Health simplifies our understanding of why we get sick. Which essentially boils down to toxins and an unhealthy gut.

At first I would use this knowledge to understand how to help patients attending my musculoskeletal clinic. I began to realise that chronic aches and pains, fibromyalgia, fatigue, painful osteoarthritis are all conditions that can be explained by low grade chronic inflammation, an unhealthy gut and toxins.

As I treated people with these conditions, I saw that their other conditions such as irritable bowel syndrome (IBS), raised blood pressure, raised cholesterol, skin conditions and constipation would also improve. Patients would then tell their friends about what I was doing and very soon, I had to quit my musculoskeletal clinic because the people that were coming to see me now had all kinds of 'labels' for their disease other than just joint or muscle problems.

I also realized that over the decades, even though there are a plethora of food programmes on TV and amazing recipe books, people have lost the innate understanding about food and its relationship to the body. There was a need to educate people about health. This is why I started my website *www.doctorese.com*. During the time that I helped my children to get well, I had to learn to prepare and cook food from scratch. I had to learn to make fermented food such as Kombucha. I was greatly helped along the way by one filled with ancient wisdom, my good friend Yasuko.

I think that I was guided to meet Yasuko one winters day in Brighton at her shop, Kantenya (which incidentally is the word for a Japanese preparation of a health-giving seaweed). Yasuko taught me just about everything I know about fermenting the Japanese way. She introduced me to the rice ferment shiokoji, which transformed the way I eat and features heavily in the book. People have thanked me from the bottom of their hearts for being introduced to this simple yet extraordinary ferment. Not only does it nutritionally and microbiologically enhance the food, but it brings the most amazing umami to the most bland dishes. You'll find me using shiokoji and other ferments on my website in the webinars I have filmed in my kitchen. The desire here was to show people first-hand how simple it is to prepare and cook health-giving food. So, the website is an educational tool to teach you what you were never taught in school. I then wanted to create a book that patients could read in one go, that explains Diet to Detox in written format with more background information and gives the related recipes all in the same book. And here it is! I hope you enjoy it.

Ese Stacey

CONTENTS

INTRODUCTION

Over thirty years ago I entered the gates of St Mary's Hospital Medical School in London's Paddington as a fresh faced nineteen-year-old. I was ready to absorb all things medical in order to help people to get well again. I thought that, if someone had a medical problem, I would diagnose it, treat it, and they would get well. Little did I know that several decades and three children later I would understand so little about what truly makes us well. In fact, I would have to learn that there is a lot more to health than medicine.

My first child, Luke, was a healthy little boy until he was around nine or ten years old, when we noticed that he would get frequent sore throats. As a medic, I thought the solution for that was obvious: whip out the tonsils. It seemed I was right – when the ENT surgeon did the tonsillectomy he said they were the worst he'd seen in a while. Luke even had tonsiloliths, hard stones embedded in the tonsils. We thought we had done the right thing. But Luke didn't get better, and nor did the halitosis (bad breath) that came with the frequent sore throats and fevers.

Next up was our second child, Harry. Harry had eczema and was passing bright green poos right from birth. The poor boy screamed and scratched his way through his first few years of life, was frequently constipated, had a constantly running nose, asthma and once had a perforated ear drum. On top of that he had mild symptoms of oppositional defiance (you ask him to do one thing and his tendency was either to say no or do the opposite) and poor concentration.

You might have thought that, as two medical doctors (my husband is an anaesthetist), we would have been well equipped to help our children with these health concerns. But this could not have been further from the truth. As doctors, we had been taught to process symptoms and formulate a diagnosis. I call this the 'car model'.

The conventional way to understand health and disease is to think of the body as a car, with working parts that break down and need to be fixed, or even replaced. Conventional medicine seeks to find which part of the car is broken. This is the diagnosis. Treatment is then aimed at fixing this broken part. In the car model of sickness, in order to arrive at a diagnosis, we need to ask about the 'symptoms' that tell us which part of the car is broken. For example, the car mechanic will ask you to explain what happened just before the car broke down. Was there black smoke coming out of the exhaust or were there funny noises? You might turn the keys in the ignition and get no response. The mechanic will run through in his mind whether there is something wrong with the electrical circuitry of the car, the exhaust or perhaps the catalytic convertor.

So for Luke, we thought the answer to the sore throats was to get rid of the tonsils. For Harry's constipation, the answer seemed to be laxatives. For his asthma, inhalers. For his eczema, steroid creams. We did all of the above. But Luke continued to be fatigued and suffer sporadic episodes of worsening health and Harry's behaviour didn't improve.

The car model – the doctor taking a set of symptoms and formulating a diagnosis – was the conventional approach to sickness that I was taught at medical school and during my junior doctor years, and it was what the doctors and I applied to Luke and Harry. Except that, as is so often the case, it didn't work.

At some point during this time, a patient of mine gave me some information about homeopathy. She suggested that I might want to read up on it as it could help me to help some of my patients. I was working in general practice at that time and I knew nothing about homeopathy, so I decided to follow up on her suggestion and eventually decided to get a full general practice-level qualification in homeopathy from the homeopathic hospital in Queens Square, London. This course opened my mind to a whole new world of thought concerning health.

Homeopathy is shunned by mainstream medicine. It is based on the principal that 'like cures like'. Samuel Hahnemann, the founder of homeopathy, discovered that he could take the very substance that caused ill health such as a poison or toxin or allergen and present it to the patient in a highly diluted form and the person would recover. Mainstream medics say that, because no substance is left in the final potentised remedy, the remedy is nothing but a placebo. In fact, progress in our understanding of quantum physics and water's ability to hold memory is beginning to shed more light onto this old form of medicine.

During my course, we had a lecture from a former hospital paediatrician who talked about using homeopathy in children. I was fortunate in that this lovely lady lived near me, so I began to consult with her about Harry's many conditions. One of the first things she told me was that his constant runny nose was not a result of repeated infections but of food intolerances.

When I look back now, I realise just how little I knew about health. There I was, a general practitioner who had at that time been qualified as a doctor for ten years, not understanding a word of what she was saying. Surely if your nose is running you have cold? Babies catch lots of colds because they are meeting new viruses all the time. This is what I thought. But what she was saying was that the runny nose was occurring as a result of the body's immune reaction to something it didn't like in its environment – namely food.

The car model of health had been so ingrained in me that I, like many doctors, had been focusing on symptoms and treatment instead of getting to the root of the problem of ill health. And here she was, telling me that diet and environment were often the root cause. We are not cars.

The homeopath told me that I had to clean up Harry's gut. But what did the gut have to do with a runny nose? I was about to learn. Harry loved his morning cereal with milk, but I had to admit that I had started to notice that his nose would start running immediately after breakfast and wouldn't stop all day. The homeopath told me that the gluten and milk in Harry's breakfast were part of the problem. I still find it astounding that I was working in general practice, seeing many children day in and day out, and I didn't know this – I simply didn't know that our gut was inextricably linked to the other systems in our bodies. At the time, I'm not sure that I really believed what she was saying. But in those days, believe it or not, the internet was in its infancy, so I couldn't even check with Dr Google. I would have to give it a try.

I did what she said and cut out the cereal and milk. Low and behold, Harry's nose began to clear up! We then went through a series of homeopathic treatments and supplements, including a probiotic, over a period of eighteen months and slowly but surely Harry's eczema began to recover too, as did his asthma and his behaviour. Over time, we were then able to reintroduce gluten and milk into Harry's diet. He continued with a low level susceptibility to them, so that if he ate gluten- or milk-containing foods on a daily basis all of his symptoms would slowly come back, whereas if he just had these things occasionally it seemed that his system could manage them.

I eventually left general practice in order to pursue my dream of becoming a sports doctor and looking after athletes in elite sport. I trained at the academic department of sports medicine at the Royal London Hospital in London. At the time this was one of the only places in the world where a doctor could train to become a sports physician. Doctors came from all over the world to do the training and it was a veritable melting pot of multicultural talent. I got the chance to visit some of the great sporting venues in the UK and in the year that followed I spent time working in Sydney, Australia and with the England Woman's rugby team. I was very proud also to be appointed to the position of Senior Lecturer at the same department where I had trained. I supervised many students and many studies during this time.

Soon after this we welcomed our third child – Hannah. Hannah has Down's syndrome (Trisomy 21), which means that she has an extra 21st chromosome. Certain health problems sometimes accompany Down's syndrome which, amongst other things, include poor immunity and a poorly functioning thyroid. These features aren't present in all children but it was clear that Hannah had some of them. Her thyroid was underactive which meant that she didn't grow so well, she was very floppy and she also had a constantly runny nose.

For some people, being given the news that your child has Down's syndrome may represent a major negative, but I am, in general, a 'glass half full' person. When Hannah came along, one of my thoughts was that these health issues were due to her chromosomes, which are DNA. I started to wonder if we could in some way make an impact on the DNA.

During my student days at the department of sports medicine, I had done some research looking at bone density in athletes who stopped menstruating. During this study, I was struck by the highly restrictive diets of these athletes. I also noted that a proportion of these athletes also had underactive thyroids and were taking Levothyroxine as a replacement medicine. It was clear to me, although I couldn't prove it at the time, that diet was playing a role in, not just the lack of menstruation, but also in the poor bone density. When Hannah came along, I started thinking about how proteins work in the body. The DNA instructs RNA to make proteins, which work in the cells. Proteins are made up of strings of smaller molecules called amino acids and are important for bone and muscle development. But not only that, the small strings of amino acids, called peptides, behave as signals in the cells, commanding them to function in certain ways.

My thoughts were that, if we could get food to 'talk' to the body in a good way, then couldn't we change the way the body behaved, perhaps in partnership with the DNA? It was then that

I really set about looking more closely into how the body deals with food.

When Hannah was four years old, we decided to have an adventure and go and live in the south of France. We loved the food, especially the bread! Hannah loved it too. We would spend school holidays at home in the UK and then return to France, and as the airplane came into land, Hannah would pipe up, "Umm! Bread!" I was still learning about food then, of course, and I still am. But I noticed that in France Hannah had a runny nose, just like Harry had some years earlier. The consequences of this constant blockage to Hannah's nasal passages were becoming more and more obvious. Hannah's runny nose would affect her sleep and she would then be very tired the next day. This in turn affected her learning at school and her behaviour.

I kept looking at the runny nose and knew I needed to do something about it, but I really didn't want her to give up her beloved bread. But eventually, we made the decision as a family to get rid of the bread. We felt it wouldn't be fair for the rest of us to be eating bread if Hannah couldn't have any, so we all stopped eating it. At this point, Luke was still suffering with sporadic episodes of fatigue and sore throats and he would constantly be clearing his throat. This was due to a post-nasal drip where mucus from the sinuses and back of the nose is constantly dripping down the back of the throat. What I noticed first after giving up the bread was that within three days Luke stopped the throat clearing. Hannah's nose took about three weeks to calm down, but it did. Because of the success of removing gluten from their diet, I thought I'd better look at a trial of removing milk products like butter, cheese and yoghurt. Low and behold, Luke's fatigue improved and so did Hannah's energy levels.

Since that time the amount of research on the gut has grown exponentially and with it our understanding of how the gut works. But in spite of this, the research has been slow to spill over into mainstream medicine. At the time of writing my son, Luke, is now a fourth-year medical student. He knows more than most medical students about the importance of good gut health, but on a recent placement in gastroenterology, very little was said about the microbiome or indeed about how food affects it. In general, he has been surprised at the poor coverage of nutrition during his medical training. Thus far, he has received four lectures on nutrition (about the same as in my day), and most of that has been derogatory.

The lack of main stream knowledge about nutrition means

that, many of us are suffering from long-term ill health or complex, chronic conditions that mainstream medicine struggles to treat. And many of us are unaware that our multiple health complaints are linked to what we eat and the environment that we live in. So perhaps it is up to us to educate ourselves about our health. Back in 2009, most of my understanding came from people who were actually using food to transform their health, particularly through fermentation. After stumbling across Sandor Katz's book *Wild Fermentation,* for example, I started to make kombucha (fermented green tea). In a short while I began to see even more health gains in my children.

On our return from France, I began working in a private musculoskeletal clinic in London. This clinic was slightly atypical in that it was set up to take patients who had not been getting better in spite of some good treatments by physiotherapists, rheumatologists and orthopaedic surgeons. Patients would present to the clinic with chronic pain in their joints despite having already been given exercises, non-steroidal anti-inflammatories, injections or maybe even operations. With my new-found knowledge about the gut, I started to ask patients to remove gluten and milk and to take a probiotic, and a good number of these patients with chronic painful joints improved.

But not everyone did. My theory – that removing gluten and milk from the diet would improve the gut – wasn't working for everyone. Was there something else causing their ill health? Then I began to notice a pattern with some of these patients who didn't improve. Many of them ate oats for breakfast. I thought the same thing that you're probably thinking – oats are good for us! Why on earth would oats make you ill? I started to research oats and realised that, of course, oats don't make you ill. People have eaten oats from time immemorial. But during this course of study into oats I began to realise that it might not be the food *itself* that makes us ill, but what's been done to it. If the oats had been left in a storage facility for long periods of time they would likely be subject to growing mould. Moulds produce toxins called mycotoxins that, you guessed it, make us sick.

I then found that it's not just mycotoxins that affect food – there are other toxins that do damage to our gut too, potentially causing a range of conditions. These could range from eczema and arthritis to joint pain and cancer. What I was slowly coming to realise was that ill health starts with toxins. Toxins in our food (and our environment) have a negative effect on the gut and it's this that really makes us ill. When we look at our body like a car and try to diagnose and treat isolated symptoms, we miss the point that our ill health is more likely to have underlying causes.

Over the years I have come to realise that when we sort out these two areas – our exposure to toxins and the health of the gut – the body can recover itself. I then used this background knowledge to develop the Diet to Detox programme to help to undo the effects of toxins and restore gut health. When we understand the Hierarchy of our Health – how our body works, and the knock-on effect of diet and environment – we can understand why we really get sick.

At school we learn how to read and write and do maths, we get qualifications and may even go to university. But no one teaches us to *be well*. In this book I want to move away from the car model of health and show how we can manage our health differently.

You may have been searching the internet, looking for an answer to the question "Why am I sick?" You may have seen doctors, specialists and had various treatments. And yet you are still not well. In this book I want to not only answer that question – "Why am I sick?" – but also provide the essential roadmap for your journey back to wellbeing. I want to help you learn what you were never taught.

The Diet to Detox programme is a step-by-step journey to good health. It has helped my patients to improve from conditions like:

Eczema
Asthma
Rosacea
Acne
Rheumatoid Arthritis
IBS
Osteoporosis
Constipation
Joint Pain
Chronic Fatigue
Thyroid Problems
Fibromyalgia
Depression
Anxiety
Obesity

The Diet to Detox programme is simple, easy to follow and does not involve cutting out food groups permanently. It is about resetting and healing the gut so you can be in optimum health. In the first part of the book I want to explain what makes us sick, why the gut is so important and the role that toxins play in our health and wellbeing. In the second part of the book you will learn the three stages of the Diet to Detox programme, how to reset your gut and improve your overall health from the inside. At the end of the book you will find recipes to help you eat the right things for your health.

We are not cars. We are complex human beings with bodily systems that are all interconnected. When you look at the body as a whole, it becomes easy to understand how to make changes that will help us to stay well.

The change starts with you.

CHAPTER 1

WHY AM I SICK?

(Names and some details are changed to protect anonymity.)
Frank was in his late forties when he came to see me at the musculoskeletal clinic. He had muscle and joint problems, specifically osteoarthritis in the knees, but surprisingly, that wasn't what he wanted to talk to me about. Frank had been sent to see me because he had severe depression and had got to the point where he was suicidal.

Frank's depression had initially come on after he had been training heavily and had lost a lot of weight. It was then compounded some years later after the death of his mother after a long illness and had progressively got worse.

When Frank came to see me he had a full beard, but despite this, I could see that just above his beard – and likely underneath – he had red patches of skin. This is called Rosacea or Acne Rosacea, and dermatologists typically treat this with long-term antibiotics. Whenever I see someone with Rosacea, I immediately think of the gut. Why? Because Rosacea is the skin manifesting what is going on in the gut.

I'd first noticed that Rosacea is linked to the gut in Hannah when she was a baby. In fact, I would regularly see this in children with Down's syndrome – the rosy red cheeks with patches of dryness a little like eczema. At first, I thought Hannah's problem was just dry skin and that she needed more moisturising cream. Then I realised that when the gut got better i.e. no bloating or gas and no constipation, then the Rosacea went away. I realised that Rosacea is linked to an imbalance in the 'good' and 'bad' gut microbes, also called gut dysbiosis. The reason antibiotics help Rosacea is because, they kill off the 'bad' gut microbes. Unfortunately, the antibiotics also kill off the good bacteria too.

I noted straight away that Frank had this indirect sign of gut dysbiosis. This was a good sign, because Rosacea responds fairly quickly to dietary changes so when patients come back to see me I can see straight away if any progress has been made. The Rosacea was therefore a good starting point. If Frank had Rosacea and therefore gut dysbiosis, my next question was, "Why does he have gut dysbiosis?" I knew from experience that, although Rosacea, osteoarthritis and depression seem like very separate issues, they were probably all linked to gut dysbiosis.

Frank began to explain his history in detail. He had been a keen rower and used to train very hard, doing a number of intense runs each week to improve his cardiovascular fitness. I asked him about his route, and he told me that his runs took him past fields that were regularly sprayed with pesticides. He also told me about his hobbies, which were renovating old cars and photography. He liked to strip down cars and repaint them.

I realised that his hobby of renovating cars undoubtedly involved the use of chemicals. As well as that, in those days, photography involved developing your own photos using chemicals. And of course there were the runs, where Frank was regularly exposed to pesticides sprayed on the fields. I ordered some investigations to look more closely at Frank's gut and to see if the chemicals he had been exposed to would show up in his urine. Sure enough, the tests suggested gut dysbiosis. The chemical tests also confirmed that there were raised levels of pesticides and chemicals. This was great to know.

But what does this have to do with Frank being suicidal?

The gut is an essential part of our being. In days gone by, we relegated it to a 'food in-faeces out' machine. But it is so much more than this. Not only is the gut an immune organ in its own right, it also has intricate links to the brain, which means that our mood is affected by our gut. Of course, we intuitively know this. When we are nervous, for example, before a job interview or performance, we might have to run off to the loo. Our nervous mind is having an effect on our gut. But the reverse is also true. The gut has an impact on the brain.

Main stream medics often treat depression with serotonin reuptake inhibitors (SSRIs) like Prozac. Serotonin improves mood, concentration and learning, and SSRIs work by stopping it from being broken down and removed from the brain, so that more is left to enhance mood. But what is interesting is that only about 5% of serotonin is made in the brain. The rest – 95% – is made in the gut.

In many of the patients who come to see me with musculoskeletal problems, for which I use a diet and environment-based approach, one of the first things that improves is their mood. Even if they don't mention it at the first consultation, they will often come back and say, "My partner says I'm much happier", or that they don't feel so stressed at work. These changes in mood can happen even before their joint pain subsides, such is the influence of the gut on the brain.

So, going back to Frank, I reasoned that perhaps low serotonin levels could be influencing his mood. Perhaps his gut dysbiosis was resulting in poor serotonin production which was impacting his brain processing.

Another factor that influences mood is inflammation. I knew from the level of toxins in Frank's urine that he was probably suffering from chronic inflammation caused by an ongoing immune response to those toxins. We will explore this later.

But suffice to say, in Frank's case, inflammation coupled with low serotonin was likely having an effect on the brain. It was also a likely factor in causing the pain and osteoarthritis in Frank's knees. So, my thought process was that if I could get Frank's gut under control, his gut would produce more serotonin, he would have less inflammation and his depression and suicidal thoughts would also come under control.

I suggested that Frank follow the Diet to Detox programme and we agreed a follow-up consultation a few months later.

When Frank came back I immediately noticed that his Rosacea had improved. His mood had also improved, so that he no longer had suicidal thoughts. He did sometimes still feel low, however, and so wasn't completely better. A few months after that he sent me an email saying that he was himself surprised by how well he felt after suffering from depression for so many years. And that wasn't all. The pain in his knees had improved so much that he was considering not having the knee replacements he'd been initially advised to have.

Frank's story illustrates how important it is to deal with our health as a whole entity. When we get sick, it is often not because one thing is wrong with us. When we look closely, we can often see several symptoms that appear unrelated, but are in fact all a result of the same issue.

Frank got better relatively quickly once we treated his gut and his progress was quite linear with few ups and downs. This isn't the case for all patients and quite often the course of progress will be an upwards trajectory but with ups and downs along the way. But what Frank's story shows is that it is not enough to look at the superficial label or diagnosis. We need to find out what has made us sick in the first place. And for that we need to understand the Hierarchy of Health.

FIGURE 1 – HIERARCHY OF HEALTH

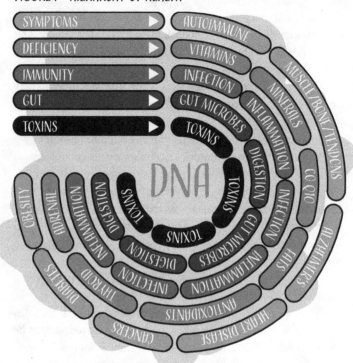

THE HIERARCHY OF HEALTH

As I've explained, most doctors – and most people – think of health along the lines of the car model I described earlier. We look at symptoms and use them to make a diagnosis before determining the best course of treatment for a particular condition. But let me present another type of analogy.

I remember once during a political election campaign in the UK, one of the politicians ran on the slogan "We are going to get tough on crime and tough on the causes of crime." This was not only a catchy slogan – it was a great idea. When a crime is committed, a good police organisation will identify who committed the crime and a good judiciary will convict the criminal and give them a suitable punishment. Whilst no-one should doubt that a good police and judiciary are essential, everyone would agree that it would be far better if the crime was not committed in the first place. Dealing with the *causes* of the crime would prevent the crime from happening. I don't want to get too political here, but I would suggest that some of the causes of crime might have something to do with emotional/social support, schooling, finances and food.

The same is true when it comes to our bodies. It is wonderful to have the correct diagnosis and even more wonderful to have a pinpointed treatment, preferably with as few side effects as possible, but wouldn't it be so much better if we could prevent the 'crime' from happening in the first place?

If you get pain in your abdomen after eating, your doctor will tell you that your symptoms are likely to be related to some kind of stomach disorder such as acid indigestion or a stomach ulcer. Using the car model of sickness, the doctor would then choose from a known list of treatments for the sick part of your body. In the case of indigestion, the treatment for increased acid production would be to give something that reduces the acid – an antacid. If this failed to fix the problem, the next step would be to do some more diagnostic tests, very much in the same way that a mechanic would analyse a vehicle. For the case of pain in the abdomen after eating, the doctor may well do blood tests looking for *H. Pylori*, a bacterial infection which is known to be associated with ulcers. If the tests are positive for *H. Pylori*, the doctor is likely to recommend a course of antibiotics to treat the ulcer. If the patient asks the doctor why they have *H. pylori*, or why they have an ulcer, the doctor is likely to say that it is because they are eating too much spicy food or even just down to bad luck. What the doctor means by 'bad luck' is bad genes. But really? Is ill health just down to a bad throw of the genetic dice?

When it comes to our bodies getting sick, preventing the crime goes beyond bad luck. Just as with crime, if we correct the social situation, we can reduce the crime. So when it comes to our bodies, what is this social situation? Well, let me present just one more analogy.

If you were to take two identical seeds and plant them in two different pots, one with good soil and one with bad soil, they will grow differently. They might have the same 'bad luck' genetics but they will grow differently in the two different types of soil. We see this with identical twins who are separated at birth and grow up in different environments – in other words, different soil. Identical twins have identical genes and yet, if they are subject to different environmental influences, they may grow and develop very differently. They may become different heights or develop completely different diseases. Researchers into genetics and disease know this and, in fact, recent studies show that genetics accounts for just 5% of disease. The rest is down to our environment. That is not to say that genes don't play any part in whether or not we develop a disease. They do. It's just that the environment is able to manipulate our genes and *switch them on or off*. This is called *Epigenetics*. So, if we view the body like a car and say that the reason it broke down was just bad luck (genes), we miss the reason why it broke down in the first place – that is, the body's environment.

I developed the Hierarchy of Health concept to show the processes that happen *before* we get sick and to show how the body is affected by its environment. It is a sea change from the way conventional doctors and many nutritionists and functional medicine practitioners view health. It is the opposite of the 'car model' of health, where the different systems of the body are treated individually.

I mentioned previously that in my practice as a sport and exercise medicine physician, I worked privately in London. Technically, all of my patients had problems with their musculoskeletal system i.e. they had bone, joint, muscle or tendon issues. I also mentioned that, the clinic I worked for was quite a specific clinic, in that it was commissioned by one of the insurance companies to try to deal with patients who were not getting better in spite of having been treated by other reputable specialists. For private healthcare in the UK, patients pay a monthly fee to the insurer and the insurer agrees to pick up the patient's bills when they see specialists. If the patient sees a lot of specialists, the insurer may end up paying out more than the patient pays in. The onus is on insurers to make sure that the books balance when it comes to patient fees coming in and payments to specialists going out. Hence, the insurers had commissioned the setup of the clinic I worked in to try to reduce the number of specialists the patient saw. A typical patient with a condition such as back pain would have seen physical therapists, orthopaedic surgeons and possibly neurosurgeons. They would have been given pain killers, exercises and possibly also injections into their back. My job was to try to make sense of the patient's condition and to help plan for a clear pathway out of the pain without using up too much more of the insurer's resources.

The insurers typically used sport and exercise medicine physicians for this because we had been trained to see the bigger picture. When looking after athletes we were trained to look beyond the joint pain and understand that wider factors impact athletes' return to their sport. What I found in the patients that came to these special clinics – patients like Frank – was that they didn't just have one problem. And herein lay the problem. The car model works well if you only have one thing wrong. But the body isn't a car and rarely is there just one thing wrong. Most of the patients I saw had more than just back pain. They might have other joints that were painful. In today's crazy medical world, this would mean that they might see one specialist for their back pain and another for their shoulder pain. Patients might be sent to see me for their knee pain and tell me that they had another appointment that same day to see a specialist that dealt with their elbow.

But it didn't stop there. These patients also often had other non-musculoskeletal symptoms such as indigestion, high blood pressure, acne, depression, an underactive thyroid, constipation, or osteoporosis. At first glance you might think that these are unrelated symptoms. You might think that it is reasonable to see a gut doctor for the constipation and an orthopaedic surgeon for your arthritis. But in the Hierarchy of Health model, just as we saw with Frank and his array of different symptoms, I can easily show you that constipation and arthritis are linked. How? Because both of these symptoms are related to chronic inflammation. And where does chronic inflammation come from? Gut dysbiosis.

Both constipation and arthritis are linked because chronic inflammation is at the root of these conditions. Research scientists are now almost unanimous in declaring that just about all chronic disease has a basis in chronic inflammation. If I focus on the gut, both the constipation and the pain in arthritis should get better. If this is the case, why don't we have 'gut clinics' instead of chronic musculoskeletal pain clinics? This is a good question and maybe in the future we will. As I've said previously, mainstream medicine always runs between twenty and fifty years behind the scientific literature, which means that we're still catching up.

So, in my musculoskeletal clinics, I began to see my patients through a gut lens and not through a muscle and joint lens. I began to suggest that my patients try a probiotic, vitamin D and vitamin K2 and a change in diet before opting for anti-inflammatory drugs, injections or surgery. I began to see results. It became clear to me that it is important to view the patient as a whole. I know, this should be obvious, right? But in medical training this doesn't happen. And it gets worse as you begin to specialise in a particular area. As specialists, we doctors are encouraged to learn more and more about our speciality. But as we do this we know less and less about how the rest of the body works. It's rather like taking a magnifying glass and looking at an elephant's toe. You really don't get a great idea about the whole elephant by just looking at its toe. If you have a rare condition, having a supra-specialist is a definite bonus. However, most people don't have rare conditions and more and more people now have more than one problem.

So what is the Hierarchy of Health and how does it explain why we get sick?

YOU AND YOUR DNA: ENERGETIC BEINGS

The Hierarchy of Health starts with you at the centre and it is represented by your DNA. Your DNA is far more than strings of genetic information. Let me try and explain more about this.

Think of yourself for a minute as an energetic being shining brightly in the universe. Did I say energetic being? If I describe a human being in these terms to conventional medics, I get an eye roll. And yet these same medics think nothing of ordering an electric heart tracing (electrocardiogram or ECG), or an electrical tracing of the brain (an electroencephalogram (EEG)). The ECG and the EEG pick up electrical charge that is given off from the heart and the brain respectively. No medic disputes this. Physics also tells us that when a charge moves through a suitable carrier (a conductor), a magnetic field is created around it. This fact was discovered in 1820 by physicist Hans Christian Ørsted. In 1826, André-Marie Ampère wrote a mathematical formula that describes the magnetic forces that occur between conductors. So, nothing particularly new there! This means that at the very least the heart and the brain produce their own biomagnetic fields.

But what if moving electric charges (or electric currents) were found in other places in our bodies? Well, of course, every cell has an electron and a proton which carry a negative and a positive charge respectively. So, we <u>are</u> electric beings! The movement of electric charge around our bodies creates a magnetic field and each organ will create its own signature field. The heart is said to create the strongest magnetic field of all the organs. Although conventional medical biology views the body as purely physical with the skin as its boundary, when we take the biomagnetic field into consideration, we must perhaps begin to view ourselves in a more expanded light. The magnetic field of the heart is measurable. As scientific instruments become more sophisticated, it seems clear that the heart's magnetic field extends far wider than a few metres around us. In his book, 'Energy Medicine', James L Oschman states

The biomagnetic field of the heart extends indefinitely into space. Every heartbeat produces an electromagnetic field that propagates into space at the speed of light, 186,000 miles per second'.

As a medical student and junior doctor, we were never taught anything about the electromagnetic activity of the heart. And yet the science has been with us for quite some time. In 1831 English chemist and physicist Michael Faraday and an American scientist called Joseph Henry discovered that magnetic fields could cause currents to flow through conductors. This is called electromagnetic induction or Faraday's Law.

I interpret this to mean that we, as electromagnetic energetic beings, have the ability to cause current to flow in anything that can conduct electricity. A coiled wire that carries electrical charge will create a magnetic field. In the human body think of the helical (or coiled) DNA. Proteins in our cells are also coiled. These too produce a magnetic field. The higher the number of coils, the more powerful the induction. Many people will have heard about pulsed electromagnetic (PEMF) devices which induce current to flow through injured tissues. PEMF type devices have been used for some time to assist in the healing of fractures. Well, it would seem that our own bodies work in the same way. The heart's magnetic fields induces pulses of charge that are carried by the blood stream around the body.

So, our bodies carry electromagnetic significance. The magnetic field of the heart has been shown to form a particular shape called a toroid. A toroidal shape is rather like a doughnut (forgive me). The central part of the doughnut is the heart and energy flows up and around the body in a continuous flow. To be well, is to maintain this perfect toroid, which in turn requires that you are subject to minimal interference.

But the problem is, we *do* experience interference. This comes from our environment around us as well as the environment within us (both physical and non-physical such as conscious and subconscious thoughts and emotions). This interference is the first layer in the Hierarchy of Health. But the important thing to remember is that **you are at the center of your health.**

THE TOXINS LAYER

The first layer in the Hierarchy of Health describes the 'interference' that we are exposed to day in, day out. We call these toxins. As we'll see in chapter 4, toxins can be from food or the way it was stored, from electromagnetic devices, from the air or even from our mental, emotional and spiritual state. The point is, these toxins have an effect on our DNA and cells.

Let me use another analogy. Imagine that in order to build a brand new cell, our enzymes and proteins are waiting for a particular sound frequency or song, say, 'Singing in the Rain'. The molecules are waiting for a particular vibratory frequency or signal before they start building the cell. But what happens if instead of 'Singing in the rain' they get 'I'm dreaming of a white Christmas'? This may mean that instead of a building a new cell, 'I'm dreaming of a white Christmas' may signal the demolition of the cell! This can be what happens when toxins become associated with either the DNA or cellular processes, they alter the cells vibratory frequency or song. These interfering toxins will cause interference in our electromagnetic signalling and so disrupt our cellular and body function. The understanding that we are energetic beings and hence can be controlled by energetic forces cannot be under-estimated. Medicine in the future will rely much more heavily on this understanding.

So can toxins in our environment explain why we get sick? I personally think that toxins play a big role in ill health and yet doctors are not taught about how toxins enter the food chain or how toxins in our environment impact our health.

Toxins have a direct action on the gut. Studies show that toxins cause damage to the gut lining cells, which is then likely to cause inflammation. Damaging the gut lining cells also means that toxins can pass directly from the gut into the body, where they can accumulate in organs and tissues. This can do direct harm to the DNA. When toxins bond to DNA they are called *DNA adducts*. When the toxin is stuck to the DNA it alters its function, in a bad way. As we are exposed to environmental toxins on a daily basis, most of us are likely to have at least one DNA adduct. When I assess my patients with chronic conditions, they usually have 2 or 3. These adducts are likely to have a major impact on long term health. The presence of multiple DNA adducts has been shown to be associated with some cancers, especially when coupled with chronic inflammation (1)

THE GUT LAYER

The second layer in the Hierarchy of health is the gut layer. For a long time conventional medicine believed that the gut's chief role was to digest food. However, we've known for some time that the gut does much more than that. In the 1800s, Nobel prize winner Elie Metchnikoff speculated about the importance of gut microbes in maintaining health. Metchnikoff noted that Hungarian peasants who drank sour milk daily, lived long lives. He surmised that the longevity was due to health-giving bacteria in the milk. Conventional medicine has only just recently begun to take notice of probiotics even though Elie Metchnikoff's work inspired further research into the gut and its relationship with microbes.

In a healthy mature large intestine (colon), we have trillions of micro-organisms living in a happy beneficial relationship with our intestinal cells. There is just a single layer of intestinal cells that separate the inside of the gut (the gut lumen) from the inside of our bodies.

Having a good profile of microbes that reside in the lumen will protect the lining cells of the gut. The lining cells should be tightly packed together with no gaps, and what is allowed into our bodies such be tightly regulated, a bit like having a customs terminal at passport control. Molecules that are allowed in have to go through proper channels and shouldn't be allowed to sneak around the sides of the customs desk.

In other words, the tight junctions between the gut lining cells should prevent passage of 'foreign' material into our body. They act as a barrier, preventing passage of unwanted material.

FIGURE 2 – GUT LINING CELLS

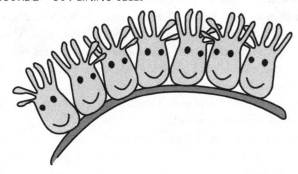

When we have a harmful profile of gut microbes (as mentioned previously this is called gut dysbiosis), the junctions between the gut lining cells are damaged, causing a breakdown in the barrier. This is where the term 'leaky gut' comes from – the gut is literally allowing foreign material through the gut lining and into our bodies. To see why this becomes a problem, we need to look at the next layer in the Hierarchy of Health.

FIGURE 3 - LEAKY GUT

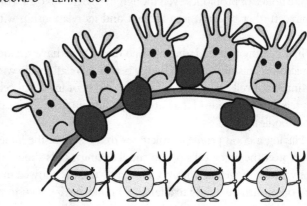

THE IMMUNITY LAYER

When foreign material escapes into the body through the gap junctions in our gut lining, they are met by our immune cells. In the image you can see the dark grey blobs of foreign material being met by the heavily armed immune cells. I call them Ninja peas because, when my husband first saw my drawings of them, he called them that. It's also easier to categorise them like this rather than to describe the different types of immune cells, so from now on that's what I will call them: Ninja peas. These Ninja peas pick up the fact that foreign material has passed through the gut wall and go into attack mode by engulfing the foreign substance. (Incidentally, it was Elie Metchnikoff who first described these Ninja immune cells, calling them phagocytes. Phagocytosis means to engulf.)

But what are the foreign materials? Basically, they are anything that is big enough to get through the gap in the gut lining illegally, stimulating an immune response. Most of us are familiar with foods that can stimulate an allergy or intolerance, such as milk or gluten. However, even small microbes readily breach the barrier, as well as particles from inhaled substances such as chemicals from perfumes or car exhaust fumes. Whatever it is, the immune cells respond by trying to engulf and dispose of the foreign material. In doing this they create inflammation which is the natural result of an immune response.

So the gut is an immune organ. But what do I mean by that? When we hear the word 'immunity', we often think of infections. Our immune cells do indeed help us to fight infections. However, they do more than that. They are also intricately linked to inflammation. Think of the inflammation that occurs if we injury ourselves. There is usually redness, swelling and pain. These reactions are actually orchestrated by the immune cells. The same types of reactions go on inside of our body as well. Take the case of hardening of the arteries (also called arteriosclerosis) that might lead to a heart attack or stroke. One theory behind how this forms says that an initial 'injury' to the blood vessel triggers the immune cells to create an inflammatory response (once again, think redness, swelling and silent pain).

The inflammatory response occurring in the injured blood vessel forms part of a whole cascade of events which attempts to heal the initial injury in the artery. This is a normal response, but if it continues and continues with no stop point, the blood vessel becomes more and more narrow and hardened until blood flow is restricted. As well as this hardening and narrowing process, some of the initial hardened plaque of inflammation can break off and get lodged in distant points which might then form a distant blockage. If this blockage occurs in the brain it would result in a stroke.

Gut dysbiosis or 'leaky gut' means that the gut no longer acts as a good barrier to prevent the entrance of microbes into the body. The gut isn't supposed to let microbes come through into our bodies and when it does, this triggers the immune cells to respond to this breach in the barrier. They respond rather in the same way as they do to an 'injury' in the blood vessel I've just described. In fact, the immune cells respond in this way not just to microbes that breach the gut barrier but also to anything that they don't recognise as normal. The immune cells will view toxins, like pesticides and chemicals, as 'alien invaders' and will try to engulf these intruders and eliminate them to prevent them from damaging our DNA and cellular mechanisms. The by-product of doing this job is inflammation.

Inflammation isn't always bad. It can be part of a normal signalling process that tells the body what to do next. Inflammation tells the body that an injury or 'invasion' has occurred. The body then sets up the correct response to deal with the anomaly and then returns back to normal. Imagine, though, if we always have 'leaky gut' and the immune cells are always 'on duty' and never get a break. Not only do we always have some form of inflammation going on, but the immune cells will also get depleted or cease to function as well as they should. This non-stop inflammation is well recognised by gut researchers, who call it low-grade chronic inflammation.

Once inflammation is created in the body, and once that

inflammation becomes chronic, the body must spend many of its resources trying to combat the inflammation. And inflammation is at the root of many conditions of ill health. Why? Because once the body can no longer cope with the chronic inflammation, we start to see deficiencies in our cellular systems.

THE DEFICIENCY LAYER

Whilst toxins, dysbiosis and chronic inflammation by themselves can cause direct harm to our body, this may be compounded by nutritional deficiencies. The 'deficiency layer' of Hierarchy of Health occurs largely because of the body's attempts to deal with the layers that have gone before. When the body is dealing with chronic inflammation, not only does it use more resources such as vitamins, minerals and hormones, but it also (because of gut dysbiosis) finds it difficult to absorb the vitamins and minerals it needs to function well. It is at this point that many people start to see symptoms and undergo tests by their doctor. Their doctor subsequently finds they are deficient in, say, vitamin D, and they are told to take a vitamin D supplement. But think back to 'Crime and the causes of crime'. The vitamin D deficiency is the crime, not the *cause* of the crime.

Whilst we're on the subject of vitamin D, let me expand a little about it. When I worked in the musculoskeletal clinic in central London, my patients were multi-cultural and would often have jobs that took them to different countries. I often did an audit on my patients to analyse their levels of vitamin D. Some patients who had just come back from a hot country would say, "I can't be low in vitamin D, I've just spent three weeks in Brazil," or some similar utterance. But I would check it anyway and I would usually find their levels to be low. In fact, I found that the only patients who were not deficient in vitamin D were those who were taking supplements. People tend to think that as we live in a northern latitude and we don't get much sun, this determines why our vitamin D levels are so low. Although I won't go into great depth here (I probably need to write a whole book on it), suffice to say that sunlight isn't the only thing that impacts levels of vitamin D – inflammation does too. Time and again, what I find is that if there is chronic inflammation the vitamin D is low. The gut may just be the link between chronic inflammation and low vitamin D. An interesting study found that if you give someone probiotics, the levels of vitamin D go up *without* giving vitamin D as a supplement. Could this be because, as the probiotics help to heal the gut, there is a reduction in inflammation which allows the vitamin D to be more easily absorbed or made?

After Hannah was born and just before we went to France, I set up a small study which I called 'The Seaford Study', after the town in East Sussex, England where we used to live. The aim of the Seaford Study was to understand what nutritional deficiencies existed in children with Down's syndrome and to give supplements to correct these deficiencies. During the Seaford Study which was funded by a charity myself and my husband had started (The Hannah Trust), I found that all five children in the small study were deficient in a number of vitamins and minerals. I encouraged the parents of the children to give supplements to bring the levels of vitamins and minerals back into the normal range. The children were so deficient that at one point Hannah was taking 13 supplements, just to maintain normal levels. The deficiencies included vitamin D, vitamin B1, 2, 6, vitamin E, zinc, and magnesium, to name some common ones. Whilst in France, Hannah was still on her supplement regime. During this time, I started to question why all of the children were deficient in so many nutrients. Was this just Down's syndrome, genetic bad luck, or was there another factor that I hadn't considered? Hannah's poos were still very up and down at this point and she would be frequently constipated. This is common in children with Down's syndrome and some children need to take regular laxatives to get their bowels to open. The gluten and milk intolerances and the nutritional deficiency led me to think about the gut. Were the nutritional deficiencies happening because of poor absorption in the gut? Was the gut not absorbing nutrients because the microbes in the gut were not performing their normal protective role? I now believe this to be the case.

In my clinics, as I found in the kids with Down's syndrome, the same types of deficiencies are present. I also see that hormonal systems can be affected by toxins, dysbiosis and chronic inflammation, including the thyroid gland, usually resulting in an underactive thyroid. The toxins, dysbiosis and inflammation trio, or TDI for short, is also a common factor in adrenal fatigue. It seems that the body, in trying to deal with TDI, overtaxes and sometimes exhausts its supply of key vitamins, minerals and hormones. It is common practice amongst medical practitioners and complementary therapists to measure and find a number of these deficiencies. I started out this way too. However, just like Hannah, it can result in you needing to take an excessive number of supplements, some of which could potentially act against one another. As well as that, some of the additional ingredients used to keep the supplement stable can cause abnormal reactions. I find that once you correct TDI, the deficiencies begin to correct themselves. Hannah hardly takes any supplements now. That's not to say that I never give supplements or that supplements are never needed. I have a range of supplements of my own that I do use regularly. Rather than containing an individual component, they are in fact powdered combinations of nutrient dense anti-inflammatory foods. However, I find that as you begin to work through the inner layers of the Hierarchy of Health that deal with TDI, the need for extra help from supplements becomes less and less.

THE SYMPTOM LAYER

The outermost layer of the Hierarchy of Health is of course when more explicit symptoms start to show. You might get high blood pressure, be overweight, have osteoporosis, acid indigestion, Alzheimer's disease, diabetes or even cancer. Under the 'car model', it is at this point that you will be treated for the health condition you have been labelled with. But these symptoms exist because of what is going on in the layers beneath. There's nothing wrong with treating these symptoms of course, but they are there for a reason. They are the 'crime' not the cause of the crime. The symptoms of disease are not there because of a bad throw of the genetic dice, but because of the whole cascade that forms the Hierarchy of Health. When we start to heal the gut and the body no longer has to deal with chronic inflammation, the outer layers often fix themselves.

Because of my understanding of the Hierarchy of Health, when a patient presents to me with a list of symptoms, I know that they are often linked. For example, constipation and arthritis are linked because chronic inflammation is at the root of these conditions. So if I know that inflammation begins in the gut, by healing the gut both the constipation and the pain in arthritis should get better.

When you understand the Hierarchy of Health, it suddenly becomes easy to see how the environment that surrounds us can prevent us from being the people we were meant to be. And when we look at each of the layers separately – the toxins we are exposed to, gut dysbiosis and the inflammation this causes, nutritional and hormonal deficiencies and the symptoms that follow – we can see how healing the gut is the key to enjoying overall good health. So let's look more closely at the gut.

CHAPTER 2

THE GUT

When I was at medical school some thirty-plus years ago, when it came to how the gut works, the emphasis was on its role in the digestion of food. We were taught to ask about the colour of stools. For example, pale floating stools might indicate malabsorption of nutrients and indicate an abnormality with the gallbladder. Black stools might suggest bleeding in the gut and hence perhaps a tumour. If the patient had diarrhoea we might measure the gut flora as it was then called (it's now called microbiota). We might look for bacteria such as *Salmonella* or *E. Coli* as a cause for food poisoning-related diarrhoea for example, but nothing was mentioned about 'good microbes'. However, as I've mentioned, research knowledge about good gut microbes was not new. Some twenty years prior to my being at St Mary's hospital Medical School, there was an understanding that a normal balance of gut microbes is important for health. The following was written in a journal published in 1966, the year of my birth:

> *When the normal balance of colonic flora is upset...,*
> *there is a risk of infection with such organisms as*
> *staphylococci and Candida albicans and there is evidence*
> *that the normal flora may be an important mechanism in*
> *clearing the gut of foreign bacteria such as salmonella.*
> PROC R SOC MED. 1966 DEC; 59(12): 1243

As a junior doctor, the first medical team I was attached to specialised in the gut (gastroenterology). I worked under supervision from some pretty high-ranking professors of gastroenterology and I was able to help with the endoscopic procedures which involve putting a camera into the stomach or colon to look at the internal architecture of the gut. Some of my patients had liver disorders such as alcoholic liver disease and some required liver transplantation. St Mary's Hospital, London, was at the time, and I believe still is, a centre of excellence for gastroenterology. However, when I was working at this prestigious department, the old knowledge had been put on the shelf. For example, the physicians were researching the cause of stomach ulcers. Now, when I was working as a junior in gastroenterology, if you had a stomach ulcer and conventional prescription medicines hadn't worked, the answer was to remove that portion of the gut. Long and complex operations were performed for these poor patients, until the knowledge began to emerge that perhaps stomach ulcers could be caused by a bacteria. Further research proved this to be true and the bacteria *H. pylori* is now treated with a course of antibiotics. This discovery revolutionised gastro-intestinal surgery. No longer were long operations – with long stays in hospital – needed. Patients could be treated by their GPs with simple antibiotics. There is no doubting that this was a beneficial discovery.

When *H. pylori* was discovered, the focus was very much on a single bacteria – a single cause of ulcers i.e. the car model. This approach suggests that our bodies are naturally sterile and become infected by a single agent that must be eradicated. But of course, this isn't true. Our intestinal tract is not sterile – old knowledge has already suggested this. In the late 1800s when Elie Metchnikoff speculated about the importance of gut microbes in maintaining health, he wasn't thinking that the gut was sterile. He had noted that many people in Bulgaria, where they drink sour milk, lived to beyond 100 years old. He postulated that this might be because of the rich source of friendly microbes in the milk – the microbes we now call probiotics. Metchnikoff's work is said to have inspired the Japanese researcher Dr Minoru Shirota to produce the probiotic yoghurt drink Yakult. The idea here is that these visiting friendly bacteria enhance the work of our own resident microbes.

Why did this knowledge take so long to become mainstream, and why is it still not fully recognised today? It almost seems as though there are parallel knowledge timelines. There is one timeline for mainstream medicine, another for research science and still another for the knowledge of indigenous populations. The Bulgarian indigenous populations are said to have fermented sheep's milk in lambskins tied around their waists. Without the benefit of refrigeration, they drank this sour fermented milk out of habit and necessity. Nevertheless, its health-giving effects were of the utmost importance. Perhaps modern research should look more closely at the habits of indigenous populations. This might help current mainstream medicine in our understanding of how to be well.

A NATURAL ECOSYSTEM

It wasn't until 2008 that systematic research into our own resident microbes was initiated by the Human Microbiome Project (HMP). The project involved researchers documenting the profile of microbes found in the nose, mouth, skin, gut and urinary tract of the human body. The aim of the research was and still is to understand the importance of gut microbes in health and disease. As research into this area has grown, there has been some clarification of the terms used to describe microbes. 'Microbiota' is used as a general term to describe all micro-organisms including bacteria, viruses and yeasts. The word 'microbiome', however, describes the micro-organisms in conjunction with their genetic material. In fact, many of the stool samples that assess the gut micro-organisms will be using techniques that measure the genetic material of the microbe rather than looking at the microbe itself.

This genetic material is vitally important to the human host. In fact, a symbiotic, two-way relationship exists between us and our microbiome. It is vital to our health. However, when we are first born, our intestines are sterile with no microbiota living in us. If we are born via a vaginal route, our first encounter with microbes comes as we travel down the birth canal. After that, with cuddles and skin contact, we accept more microbes onto our skin. Over the next few years, up until the age of four, our microbial profile develops and matures. If we are born via caesarean section, we don't have as much immediate contact with maternal microbes. However, under normal circumstances, the microbial profile will still develop and mature as normal, it just may take a little longer. Breast feeding also provides a good dose of beneficial microbes.

THE HEALTHY GUT MICROBIAL PROFILE

It is clear that our microbial ecosystem has an effect on our own metabolic functioning. The gut microbes produce vitamins, fats, amino acids and other molecules that have various roles, including inflammation reduction. For example, one of our resident gut microbes is able to produce short chain fatty acids (SCFAs). You might know these as ketones, the things that give the acetone-like smell to the breath when we fast. SCFAs have a number of roles in the gut. They can help the lining cells of the gut, so strengthening the gut barrier. They can also help to resist the growth of harmful microbes such as *Salmonella*. They also pass through the gut and act as signalling molecules, giving instructions to distant organs such as the liver, the heart and the brain. One such SCFA, butyrate, is even said to help lower blood pressure. As I said in chapter 1, if I check for vitamin deficiencies in my patients, I often find that the B vitamins are lacking, especially vitamins B1, 2, 6 and 12. These vitamins seem to get used up when the patient is battling chronic inflammation. What is fascinating is that the healthy gut produces all of these vitamins all by itself, as well as folate (2). Vitamin K2 is another vitamin that is often low in the general population. It is linked to healthy bones, prevents osteoporosis and gives young-looking skin. In food it is hard to come by. The Japanese eat a vitamin K2 food called Natto, made from fermented soya beans. Natto is an acquired taste, has a distinctive smell and is stringy. But it turns out that vitamin K2 is also produced by a healthy microbiome (2).

You might have heard of a beneficial molecule that is present in oats called beta-glucan. Beta-glucan confers oats with some of their beneficial actions of lowering cholesterol, providing fibre for the gut and preventing cancer. Well, wouldn't you know it, but a healthy microbiome can also produce its own version of beta-glucan (2). This may explain why indigenous communities that eat few fruits and green vegetables can still be very healthy. Take for example the indigenous Inuit population of Greenland. Their habitat is frozen much of the year, so they don't have much chance to eat fruit and green vegetables. Although eating habits have become more westernised now, the traditional Inuit would eat raw or fermented meat and fish (3). In fact, one staple of the native Inuit diet is the contents of caribou intestines. It might sound pretty disgusting, but of course it is all full of microbes and microbial breakdown products.

As we have seen, the resident microbes in the gut also produce neurotransmitters such as serotonin, as well as other molecules such as noradrenaline, dopamine and acetylcholine, which are all made in small quantities by our resident gut microbes.

For a better understanding of the gut microbiota, we should first start with a simplistic representation of gut anatomy.

FIGURE 4 – GUT ANATOMY

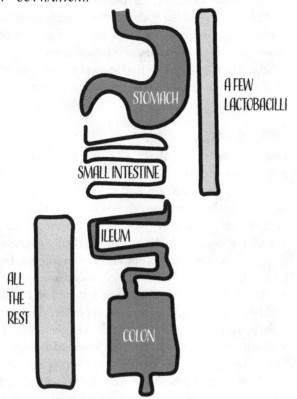

The upper (small) intestine should be relatively free from microbes. You do find a few microbes here but in general, the gastric juices should be acidic enough to keep numbers low.

In a healthy mature colon, we have trillions of microbiota living in a happy beneficial relationship with our intestinal cells. The physical abundance and diversity of the gut microbiota can have a direct effect on our health. Not only that, but the microbiome holds at least ten times more genetic material than we have in our body. This means there's more of 'them' than 'us'! Why is this important? It is important because of the phenomenon we discussed in chapter 1 called 'Epigenetics'. Epigenetics is what occurs when our genes are switched 'on' or 'off'. This means that if you possess the gene for say, diabetes, you won't necessarily develop diabetes. The gene would need to be switched 'on' for it to alter your metabolic processes. One of the things responsible for the switching 'on' and 'off' of these genes is the gut microbiome. This is enormous for our understanding of what makes us sick. If the microbiome can switch on and off our own genes, this means that many of the chronic diseases we have can be modified by modifying the microbiome.

Rather than looking at the effect of a single micro-organism, researchers have established that the effect on our genetics is driven by certain collections, or 'profiles' of microbes. A normal beneficial profile would keep us in good health. A pathogenic or 'bad' profile (i.e. gut dysbiosis) can have an epigenetic effect and make us sick.

MICROBIAL DIVERSITY IS KING

Research pioneered by the HMP reveals that microbial diversity is important for a healthy life. It can be useful to think of the microbes living in our gut rather like the kingdom of animals that live on earth. You have different types of animals and within each animal group you have different types of that specific animal. For example, in the animal kingdom, you might think of dogs, cats, and elephants. But also within the dog family you have different types of dogs. The gut microbiota are like this and are classified in a very similar manor to the animal kingdom. You could say that we have a whole world or kingdom of microbes living in our gut. The more diverse this kingdom is, the greater its ability to respond to different environmental influences. This means that the more different types of beneficial microbe there are in our gut, the healthier we are. Traditional and remote societies that eat a wide variety of natural foods have been shown to have a wide gut diversity. This gut diversity is associated with improved health when compared with highly 'developed' populations (4).

As we get older our gut microbes become less diverse. This is linked with increasing ill health. But older people with wide microbial diversity are healthier than those with narrow microbial diversity (5).

FIGURE 5 - GUT MICROBIOTA COMMUNITY

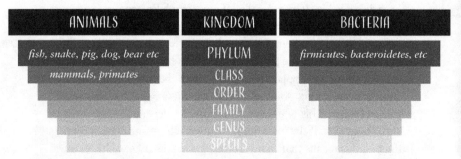

ANIMALS	KINGDOM	BACTERIA
fish, snake, pig, dog, bear etc	PHYLUM	*firmicutes, bacteroidetes, etc*
mammals, primates	CLASS	
	ORDER	
	FAMILY	
	GENUS	
	SPECIES	

FAT MOUSE – THIN MOUSE

Even in Western populations, which have narrow microbial diversification, there seem to be profiles of bacteria that can be associated with better health. You might have heard the expression 'Calories in, Calories out'. The interpretation of this statement is that the number of calories you eat will determine whether or not you lose or gain weight. However, this notion is challenged by research into gut microbial profiles. For example, researchers have found that people with obesity have a different microbiota profile than that of thin people. This means that if two people are given the same number of calories, but one person has an 'obese profile' and the other a 'slim profile', the person with the 'obese profile' of microbes is likely to harvest more calories from the food they eat and gain more weight than the person with the 'slim profile' of microbes, even if they are both given the same food to eat.

There is fascinating basic research to support this. Researchers looking into the gut microbiome like to use germ-free mice in their experiments. Germ-free mice have no gut microbes. They are sterile. The researchers can take microbes from mice with healthy gut profiles and insert them into the germ-free mice and study what happens to them. The process of transferring microbes (faeces) from mouse to mouse is called faecal matter transplant (FMT). In one experiment, researchers performed FMT from a normally developing mouse into a germ-free mouse. Germ-free mice are underweight, but after the FMT from a normal mouse, the germ-free mouse gains weight.

FIGURE 6 – GERM-FREE MICE EXPERIMENTS

NORMAL MICROBES   OBESE MICROBES

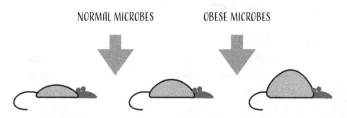

The calorie content of the mouse food is kept the same for both the normal mouse and the germ-free mouse. This means that the weight gain in the germ-free mouse is directly related to the FMT. So, far so good. Then the researchers take faecal matter from an obese mouse and transplant it into a normal weight mouse. The normal weight mouse, eating the same calories as usual, then gains weight. These fascinating experiments suggest that there's more to obesity than 'Calories in, Calories out'.

Then the researchers go one step further and take a 'slim' microbial profile from a slim mouse and transplant it into the obese mouse and, low and behold, the obese mouse, eating the same calories as previously, now becomes slim. I cannot help but think that the 'microbiome pill' will be coming to pharmacy near you shortly – in fact, a glance at Google Patents reveals that several have already been proposed.

And this suggestion is not so far-fetched. Hospital researchers have used FMT to treat resistant diabetes. They have transplanted a 'good' non-diabetic microbiota profile into a severely diabetic individual and 'switched' off their diabetes. Hospitals in the UK are beginning to go through the necessary regulatory steps to start conducting FMTs on patients with severe diabetes. Some private health clinics already offer this FMT therapy. It can seem as though FMT is a new thing but actually it is as old as the hills. Traditional societies have been known to use this technique for the treatment of sick people way before we started writing about it in research articles.

Knowing what we do about the importance of the microbiota profile, we might easily want to search for conditions that occur as a result of a faulty gut. This is how scientific research has approached the topic of gut dysbiosis. The focus is often on a particular profile of microbes with the aim of defining which disorder matches the abnormal profile. The objective being, to be able to create that 'microbiome pill for the ill'. However, this is simply returning to the car model of health. The Hierarchy of Health – the understanding that there are layers of health and that each one cascades to the next – challenges this conventional view.

WHY DOES THE GUT GO WRONG?

So why do more and more people have more than one health problem? My theory about this is that chronic inflammation in the general population is worsening. When I first started working as a doctor, I mainly saw either children with acute illnesses or older people with multiple problems (also called multi-morbidity). However, as the years progressed, I began to see more and more younger people presenting with multi-morbidity. It could be a joint problem or a tendon problem that just didn't want to get better and this might be combined with difficulty losing weight or fatigue or work stress.

I remember one particular case in a young woman called

Stella, who was in her late twenties. She had had a shoulder injury that lingered on, despite having had some good physiotherapy to work on strengthening the correct muscles. She also said that she had a vague pain across her back and shoulders. She described it as something between a pain and a stiffness. It would vary in intensity from day to day. She also struggled to get out of bed in the mornings due to extreme fatigue, she felt her thought processes were often muddled and she wasn't entirely happy with her job. This type of pain coupled with fatigue, brain fog and anxiety are fairly common in my patients. If I drill down, I will also find that they may have issues with their gut such as bloating, indigestion and constipation. This type of presentation is also typical for fibromyalgia. Fibromyalgia is a condition where all of these seemingly disparate symptoms are lumped under one label. Researchers don't have a specific 'car model' cause for it. A decade or more ago, it was something that I rarely saw and if I did, it was usually in women in their fifties. Yet now, even the term 'brain fog' seems to be commonplace. When I trained thirty years ago, this term didn't exist.

I asked Stella to remove the 'culprit foods' (I'll explain what these are in chapter 6) and to take a probiotic, vitamin D and K2. Her symptoms were greatly improved in just a few weeks. However, Stella told me that she really began to believe that it was food affecting her condition when, after work one day, she had no proper food in the house and decided to have a bowl of cereal with milk. The next day she woke up in a lot of pain, with worse brain fog and fatigue than before. She felt as though she had gone back to square one or even worse. The re-introduction of culprit foods after a period without them, saw the return of symptoms, suggesting that toxins and gut dysbiosis and therefore inflammation, were a major part of the problem.

After a number of years working with patients presenting with chronic muscle and joint conditions, I would give talks to colleagues and the general public and gradually I began to see patients with different types of presenting conditions and not just muscle and joint conditions. I've already spoken about Frank who came to see me with depression and suicidal thoughts. I have seen patients with constipation and osteoporosis, with asthma and hay fever. The fibromyalgia type of presentation is probably the most common. After many years of seeing patients with different types of labels, I've come to realise that whatever affects the gut affects us. I believe that we all have some degree of leaky gut. After all, researchers state that the aging process is caused by chronic inflammation and chronic inflammation is caused by a leaky gut. The wellbeing of our gut really does affect our general health and wellbeing. But as I explained in chapter 2, what is important to understand is that inflammation is an immune response (Ninja peas). The next chapter looks at the Ninja peas in more detail.

CHAPTER 3

THE GUT AND THE IMMUNE SYSTEM

When my second son Harry was born, he cried – a lot. My poor son would cry and cry because his skin was itchy, and when I bathed him the crying got worse. Initially, I thought that it was because he wasn't used to the water, so I bathed him even more. It breaks my heart to think about this period now. A few months after he was born, I noticed red patches appearing behind both knees. For weeks, I couldn't work out where these patches were coming from. Then, one night when I was checking on him, I found my answer. Harry's skin was so uncomfortable that he would use the nail on his big toe to reach the back of his opposite knee to scratch his itchy skin. My poor baby boy had to turn into a contortionist to reach the itchy spots behind his knees. It was this big-toe-facilitated scratching that was causing the red patches.

Harry's eczema continued to get worse until we had to wrap his arms and legs in bandages. We would need to put a layer of steroid cream and emollient lotion on the skin, then a layer of bandages, then more cream on top of the bandages, followed by a final layer of bandages. This was very soothing for him but he did look a little odd. We also had to bathe him in potassium permanganate. This is a purple crystalline powder that you add to the bath water. Again, it is very soothing, but the colour changes from purple to brown and everything that touches it becomes brown. We had a lot of brown towels.

As well as the eczema, Harry also had a constantly running nose and asthma. The asthma required preventer (steroid) inhalers as well as reliever inhalers. His skin was very pale and he also had a bloated tummy and constipation. He was extremely picky with his food and would 'react' to certain foods. My husband and I used to show people that if we even let Harry sniff orange squash he would instantly become hyperactive and start running around the room.

As we've seen, as doctors we simply thought that Harry's issues were bad-luck genetics. It was only once I started to see a homeopath and she started to explain to me about food intolerances that I began to understand how the gut fitted into Harry's story.

The homeopath had told me that homeopathy doesn't work if

the 'terrain' is not healthy. By 'terrain', she meant the gut and the nutrient status of the body. She had suggested some investigations on Harry which pointed to multiple nutrient deficiencies and gut dysbiosis. I embarked upon some dietary changes for Harry, eliminating some 'culprit' foods, taking supplements and giving him a probiotic. Slowly but surely, Harry began to recover. The bloating and constipation settled. His hyperactivity settled. His asthma went away. His eczema went away. Within reason he can now eat most foods. And thankfully Harry is no longer fearful of water – in fact, he is now a top level swimmer.

By now you might understand that Harry's symptoms can all be explained by leaky gut. I mentioned in the previous chapter about leaky gut or gut dysbiosis. Gut dysbiosis describes a harmful profile of gut microbes that damage the intestinal layer of gut cells. This damage ruins the gap junctions in between cells that serve to create the gut barrier wall that prevents unnecessary passage of harmful molecules. But what happens once these toxins have entered the body through the gut? How does that make us sick?

NINJA PEAS

Thus far, I've explained how gut dysbiosis or the leaky gut comes about. The harmful alien molecules present in our food help to create this situation. Food is not the only place to find these gate crashers. But we'll stick to food for now. Once the harmful aliens have gained access to our body, through the permeable gut lining, they are immediately met by our immune cells.

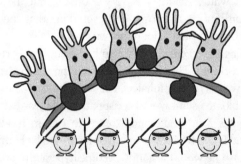

As you know, I call these cells the Ninja peas. It's also a helpful name because the subject of immune cells is quite complicated and if I started talking about innate immunity, cellular immunity and humoral immunity, you probably wouldn't go to the next page. So, I call them all Ninja peas.

When harmful alien molecules pass through the gut, it is the job of the Ninja peas to recognise and deal with the aliens. This means either swallowing them up, breaking them down or transforming them into something less harmful. This process takes time and energy and produces by-products and debris. These by-products and debris is what causes inflammation. Let me give you an example.

When a virus gains entry into the body, either through the mouth or nose, this harmful alien passes through the mucosal layer in the nose or mouth. This is similar to the mucous layer in the small and large intestines. After gaining entrance, the Ninja peas will spot this alien and try to deal with the virus so that it cannot replicate and do damage to the body. But in the process of engulfing, breaking down or transforming the virus, the Ninja peas produce by-products such as cytokines, and debris such as free radicals, or broken down bits of cell wall. It is the inflammation from these by-products and debris that is responsible for your cold or flu symptoms. It is the by-products that cause the shivering, aching, and fever that go with a cold or flu, not the virus itself.

In this case, the harmful alien invasion is due to a virus that causes an infection, but the exact same process happens for invasions that are not due to infection but are due to toxins from your food. To borrow (or butcher) from Rudyard Kipling's poem 'If' – the Ninja peas treat both imposters just the same.

Any invasion, whether it be infectious or not, is treated in the same manner by our immune system. Our ever-vigilant Ninja peas respond by dealing with the attack and, in the process, produce some inflammation. This means that immunity and inflammation are inextricably linked, and that is why in the Hierarchy of Health I call the third layer the immunity layer, because the Ninja peas are the central players that deal with infection and both create and deal with inflammation.

CHRONIC INFLAMMATION

Researchers state that low-grade chronic inflammation is the underbelly of most chronic illness. And yet this silent, low-grade inflammation that hurts our body, accelerates aging and makes us feel unwell is just not recognised by mainstream medicine. Many people who go to their GP with a chronic health complaint will find that the GP will routinely measure this inflammation. They commission the standard blood tests for inflammation – the erythrocyte sedimentation rate test (ESR) and the c-reactive protein test (CRP). People with an acute viral infection, like influenza will have a raised ESR, indicating that the Ninja peas are attacking the virus. A chronically raised CRP on the other hand, representing chronic inflammation, is linked to the diseases of western living, like diabetes, heart disease, raised cholesterol and stroke.

However, sometimes chronically ill people, particularly those with chronic fatigue and fibromyalgia, do not have a raised ESR *or* CRP. When these and other standard blood tests that look for anaemia, liver and kidney function are normal, the GP will more often than not declare that all is well. And yet, the patient is still *un*well. Why?

The ESR and CRP tests are in fact indirect markers of inflammation. To spot chronic inflammation, we need to understand how immune cells behave. As I mentioned, immune cells are not only responsible for creating inflammation, but they are also responsible for clearing up the inflammatory 'mess'. Immune cells also help in the process of building up and breaking down of cells. This process is called cell turnover. Cell turnover is a natural process that helps to keep our body refreshed and regenerated. When inflammation is present, the immune cells will deal with this situation by either regenerating new cells or by accelerating the process whereby natural programmed cell death occurs (apoptosis). Apoptosis is key to our understanding of what makes us get old.

But if inflammation is the cause of most chronic disease, including aging, and the Ninja immune cells play a critical role in this process, what happens when the Ninjas get sick?

If the Ninjas can't regenerate our cells properly or apoptosis doesn't happen, the sick cells that should have died or been made new, go rogue. The normal building up and breaking down becomes dysfunctional, and this is how we get tumours. Tumours are growths or clumps of cells and, to a certain extent, we have this process happening all the time. The Ninja peas, act as immune surveillance cells, monitoring and controlling this situation. The body uses its nutrient resources such as vitamins, minerals, amino acids, proteins and hormones, to do this. But when the immune system is overwhelmed, tumours may then be allowed to get completely out of control. When they get to a critical level and enough of them have gone rogue, we have symptoms such as fatigue and weight loss and see physical signs such as a lump.

When ESR and CRP tests come back normal, but the patient is still suffering symptoms, I delve deeper. And when I measure cell turnover instead of these indirect markers, I can then 'see' the inflammation. Of course, cell turnover is also an indirect sign but it's a marker of Ninja activity as they try to break down damaged cells and build up new ones. The more serious the inflammation, the higher the values I see for the cell turnover. I don't know for sure why the ESR and CRP are often normal in chronic fatigue and fibromyalgia patients. It's as if chronic fatigue and fibromyalgia are representative of a type of 'cold' inflammation, whereas someone with rheumatoid arthritis and swollen joints will have 'hot' inflammation and both ESR and CRP are raised. The point is that there is a link between immunity and inflammation – and it all starts with the first two layers of the Hierarchy of Health: toxins and the gut.

So why are we seeing more and more people with chronic ill health? I can only conclude that chronic conditions are increasing because our exposure to toxins is increasing. This is not generally accepted by mainstream medicine because we are not taught that toxins can be a 'silent' cause of chronic ill health. But they are. And in the next chapter we'll find out why.

CHAPTER 4

TOXINS

Elena was in her fifties when she came to see me but she looked much older. She was quite dishevelled – she was carrying lots of bags, she mumbled a lot and she would constantly spit into a tissue. Elena was convinced that she had mercury poisoning from her metal fillings. Now, at this point in my career I knew nothing about toxins, but I had completed my medical homeopathy training. In homeopathy, when we learn about a particular remedy, we learn about a symptom picture or character that goes with the remedy. The other foundation principle discovered by Dr Hahnemann, the father of homeopathy was that 'like cures like'. This means that the same substance that caused the problem or condition can be used to cure the problem, but the curative remedy would be in the diluted potentised form.

The understanding of 'like cures like' was important for my understanding of what was bothering Elena. In homeopathy, mercury toxicity has a particular description. You might remember the nervous, confused character of the Mad Hatter in Lewis Carroll's 1865 book *Alice's Adventures in Wonderland*. In fact, the term 'mad as a hatter' was coined before *Alice in Wonderland* was written and described the character of hat makers who used mercury to turn animal fur into felt. The long-term accumulation of mercury in the body would result in psychiatric symptoms: confusion, slurred speech, hair loss, tremors, abdominal pain, diarrhoea and hypersalivation. I had to admit that Elena's characteristics and the homeopathic symptom picture for mercury seemed to fit together.

At the time, as I was so new to homeopathy and to the idea that toxins could cause disease, I referred Elena on to a more experienced practitioner. Of course, there is a lot of debate about whether or not metal fillings, which are made up of an amalgam containing mercury and other metals, really do cause ill health. As I mentioned previously, the car model looks for a single cause of ill health, whereas the Hierarchy of Health usually finds more than one contributing factor that disturbs the body's equilibrium. But it made me think that perhaps toxins are more common than we think as a cause of ill health.

I now believe that toxins play a big role in ill health, and yet doctors are not taught about how toxins enter the food chain or how toxins in our environment impact our health. Before we look at individual toxins, let's first remind ourselves how toxins make us sick.

DNA AND EPIGENETICS

In the mid-2000s the health market became flooded with biotechnology companies offering DNA checks. The idea was that if you know your DNA, you know what diseases you will get. However, as I've mentioned previously, having a gene for a disease doesn't necessarily mean that you will develop the disease. You might have heard of the BRCA gene, which is associated with an increased risk of developing breast and ovarian cancer. If you carry this gene, your risk of developing these cancers can be as high as 8 in 10, or 80%. And yet the risk that comes with carrying the BRCA gene hasn't always been this high. It used to be around a 1 in 4 chance, or 25%. If the gene was a highly important factor in whether or not you developed these cancers, wouldn't the risk just stay the same? What caused the risk to go up? The answer is inflammation. Everything that reduces inflammation would reduce your risk of getting these cancers, and anything that increases inflammation would increase your risk of getting these cancers. This is because, although the gene is the processing pathway that tells you which disease you will get, it can be switched 'on' and 'off'. I explained previously that this switch is called *Epigenetics*.

The same is true for non-cancer conditions. You may have the gene for high blood pressure or some other chronic condition, but this doesn't mean that you will go on to develop this condition. Your genes are *not* your destiny. In fact, many of the biotechnology companies that came with great fanfare to test our DNA, no longer exist. Why? Because the gene couldn't predict our lives.

Of course, the gene does still play a role, as it determines which disease you get – but only if the gene is switched on. So, the logical next question is, what switches the gene 'on' and 'off'? This again, does not follow the car model. There isn't one single factor that switches the gene 'on' and 'off'. It's a combination of things. Anything that causes inflammation will have the potential to flip the switch. Toxins, by virtue of the fact that they cause inflammation, are important here. But as we have seen, toxins also do something other than cause inflammation. They can form bonds with DNA called DNA adducts. When the toxin is stuck to the DNA as an adduct, it has the ability to flip the 'bad' switch and turn a particular gene on.

As mentioned above, toxins may also affect health via a direct action on the gut. Toxins will cause direct damage to the gut lining cells, causing more inflammation and allowing direct passage of toxins from the gut into the body, where they can accumulate in organs and tissues and do direct harm to the DNA.

So where do toxins come from? And how can we avoid them?

WHERE DO TOXINS COME FROM?

As mentioned before, we are bombarded by toxins all the time. There are toxins that cause air and water pollution, toxic chemicals food packaging, and toxins in beauty products such as creams, shampoos, conditioners and cosmetics. Toxins can be chemicals like pesticides and insecticides that are used to spray animals and foods, or chemicals used in soft furnishings such as cars, sofas and curtains. They could be heavy metals found in foods, make-up, tooth fillings and tattoos, or mould or mycotoxins from water-damaged buildings or stored and dried food. My story about Elena and homeopathy makes for an interesting story, but is there really evidence of a link between environmental toxins and serious health conditions?

Let's think about some of the toxins we already know about. We now know that smoking cigarettes can lead to lung cancer. This is a known and accepted link. When we think of tobacco smoke we naturally think of nicotine, but Cancer Research UK tell us that burning cigarettes release at least 5000 different chemicals, of which 70 can cause cancer (6). The diverse cancer-causing chemicals in cigarette smoke include chemicals derived from petrol such as Benzene, benzo(a)pyrene and 1, 3 butadiene. But cigarettes also contain heavy metals such as chromium 6, arsenic and cadmium, preservatives such as formaldehyde and, as if that wasn't enough, radioactive substances such as polonium-210 and beryllium. Tobacco and tobacco smoke also contain not only mycotoxins, but bacteria and bacterial toxins (7). Tobacco smoke has even been found to contain pesticides. This diverse array of toxins in cigarette smoke combines to irritate the lungs and cause inflammation, and chronic inflammation promotes the growth of harmful microbes. Add to this heavy metals and plastics from other sources, and you have the perfect environment to encourage rogue cell turnover.

Tobacco smoke is a good example of the different types of

toxins that can affect our health. But when I measure toxins in my patients, whether they smoke or not I find toxins from the same categories occurring all the time. These are:

Heavy metals
Mycotoxins
Pesticides
Plastics

Take Jenny, for example. Jenny was seventeen years old and a promising young track and field athlete when she came to see me. However, over a one to two-year period, she had become more and more fatigued and had developed low level pain in her muscles. The situation got so bad that eventually she had to stop going to school. She could manage around two hours of school work per day before becoming exhausted. She also had to stop her beloved sport. Jenny also had some gut symptoms. She would have bouts of diarrhoea then sometimes constipation. Certain foods would 'irritate' her stomach and cause pain when she ate.

One of the things that struck me when I saw Jenny was that she wore a lot of make-up. Of course, many people wear a lot of make-up – that's not unusual. When I asked about the make-up, Jenny's mum told me that Jenny had worn heavy make-up every day since she was fourteen years old. I then asked about other household 'culprit' chemicals. Jenny told me she liked to wash her hair a lot and would go through one to two bottles of shampoo and conditioning lotion *per week*. Now, perhaps you wouldn't automatically think that wearing make-up and washing your hair could be a source of toxins, but it is. The skin absorbs chemicals and the chemicals get taken up into our blood stream. Some of the chemicals will get dropped off into various organs and tissues along the way. I once spoke to a scientist who worked in the pharmaceutical field looking at mathematical modelling to determine what happens to the chemicals that we put on our skin. To my horror, he told me that a good many end up in our brain. The body, of course, will try to deal with the toxins, using the liver to try to transform them into less harmful substances. This process is called biotransformation. The liver and the gut are intimately linked and the blood passing through the liver also passes through the gut in a process called entero-hepatic circulation (EHC). The EHC means that toxins moving around the body, whether they were inhaled or put on your skin, will eventually end up in the gut. These toxins will harm the balanced profile of beneficial microbes as well as directly harming the gut lining cells. The injured leaky gut then promotes inflammation, as we saw in chapter 2.

I told Jenny that I thought that her symptoms might be coming from the toxins in her self-care items, and we measured the toxins that the body was expelling via urine tests. Normally, when I do the urine tests, I will find four or five toxins that contribute to the body's dis-ease. With Jenny we found *seventeen* different chemicals, toxins and metals.

So where exactly had all these toxins come from? Well, the greasy part of make-up contains petrol or plastic derivatives. Of these there may be several different types of chemical, each giving a different property, texture or feel to the cosmetic. The colours in the cosmetics can come from heavy metals. Think of the reds, blues, greys, greens and blacks in make-up. Many of these colours are heavy metals. And what about the fragrance in cosmetics, shampoos and lotions? Apparently, the term 'fragrance' can represent a mix of 3000 different chemicals (8).

And even fragrance-free cosmetics can contain chemicals. A study performed by Health Canada found that 100% of cosmetics contain nickel and 90% beryllium (8). Ninety-six percent contain lead. There is currently no safe level of lead. Other metals, such as arsenic, cadmium and mercury, were also present. Does it remind you of tobacco smoke?

I advised Jenny to rethink her cosmetic, shampoo and conditioner use. I asked her to try and find non-toxic alternatives and perhaps to go make-up free for a while. I also advised her to follow my Diet to Detox protocol to give the gut a chance to heal. Jenny had been unwell for a few years, but within a few weeks of making the changes she started to feel well enough to go to school. Then, after another short while, she began to do sport again.

Jenny's and Elena's stories show that toxins can enter the body from the things we put on and in our bodies. But toxins can also have built up from before we were even born.

THE MULTI-GENERATIONAL EFFECT

I often ask my patients where they grew up. It might not seem relevant to someone who is suffering ill health in their fifties or sixties, but I do it because I know that toxins can build up over a period of decades. For example, as a child they may have been exposed to pesticides as a result of living near fields that were regularly sprayed. This could have an effect on their gut even many years later.

We must also consider that the exposure to toxins might have occurred before they were conceived, i.e. in their mother. In fact, the epigenetic switch may have been flipped several generations before the person in the present day gets the disease. For example, researchers have shown that a grandmother being exposed to pesticides would have the rheumatoid arthritis gene switched on and this genetic position would be passed on to her offspring. Her offspring can then pass it on to the next generation, and so on (9).

I have also found that toxins themselves can be passed from one generation to the next. A friend of mine who is a doctor came to me after having suffered with ill health and fatigue for a number of years. Both her parents were dentists. When we checked her levels of toxins we found high levels of mercury found in dental fillings. Of course, there may have been other sources of the mercury, but this generational mode of transmission has been well documented in the environment and the animal and fish food chain.

I also ask my patients if they grew up or live by a busy road. Air pollution as a direct cause of death was given national prominence recently when the *Daily Mail* newspaper ran an article about the death of a nine-year-old girl who suffered with asthma (10). The girl lived on a busy road in south London. Her hospital visits were correlated with local spikes in air pollution and the death was directly attributed to air pollution. The article also points out that the number of deaths associated with air pollution is on the increase. This is a curious finding: London no longer lives under the black smog of the 1950s and 60s and yet air pollution is causing more ill health than ever before. Could it be that our bodies are already primed by other toxins, making us more susceptible to the toxins in the air?

MOULDS

Toxins are hardly ever present by themselves. There is usually a mix of toxins plus infections or inflammation. However, mould and mycotoxins often give familiar symptoms. Mould and mycotoxin symptoms are familiar not because they fit a set pattern but because they can be so odd. So odd, in fact, that mainstream medics often label the person as mentally unwell. Sarah was one of my first patients with mould problems. As a result of having recurrent sinusitis, her ENT surgeon in Denmark had taken tissue samples and told her she had aspergillus growing in her sinuses. Aspergillus is a fungus. Now, sinusitis as a result of a fungal infection is not uncommon. It was her other symptoms that were striking and, ever since, I look out for these types of otherwise unexplainable symptoms. Sarah told me that her symptoms would be relatively 'quiet' until around 4 pm, when she would, as she described it, have 'showers' of pain starting in her abdomen and spreading like electricity around her body. These showers of pain would continue for several hours. She would sometimes also feel as though 'things were moving around her body' – always after 4 pm.

I have since heard similar stories from patients of feelings of throbbing in different parts of their body, or 'things' moving. The symptoms are usually worse either after a meal or in the late afternoon. Now, these strange symptoms alert me immediately to the presence of mould or mycotoxins. A lot more research is needed, but I believe it is the spores that hatch in the evening that causes these symptoms. The symptoms worsening after food is likely to represent feeding time for the microbial overgrowth in the upper gut. Moulds and mycotoxins can also cause fibromyalgia-type aches and pains. An interesting study found that a cluster of workers in Finland who had moved into a new building developed joint aches and pains. Some developed classical genetic rheumatoid arthritis and others had symptoms that mimicked it. When they searched this new building, they found mould under the floorboards (11).

When I questioned Sarah about what she thought the source of the mould could be, she said that on returning back to the UK from Denmark, she searched her house and in her bedroom she found that the whole of the back of her wardrobe was covered in green mould.

So we have learnt that toxins are present in many of the chemicals that we put on or in our bodies, the environment we are exposed to and even the environment our parents were exposed to before we were born. But there is another, greater source of toxins that get direct access to the gut: our food.

CULPRIT FOODS

At the start of this book I described how, when I first stumbled on this journey into the gut, I used to ask my patients to avoid gluten and milk-containing foods. Some of the patients would respond well and their conditions would improve, but others would not, and it was then that I noticed that many of the people who did not respond, liked to eat oats for breakfast. I started to look at research articles and stumbled over an article about turkeys dying after eating mouldy peanuts. This prompted me to start looking at food contaminants, and bingo – I found that oats *are* good after all. It was the way they are stored and packaged that was the problem.

So what are the harmful alien molecules that can contaminate oats? To answer this question, let's look at what happens when oats are grown, harvested and processed.

Oats are a cereal, and they need good soil to grow in. In fact, soil itself is an important consideration that we've all but forgotten about when it comes to understanding how healthy our food is. We concentrate on what our food is sprayed with but we don't think much about the nature of the soil it is grown in. Good soil is alive! It is teaming with inter-living microbes, insects and organisms. In Rachel Carson's book *Silent Spring*, she says, "a teaspoonful of topsoil may contain billions of bacteria" (12). Bacteria in soil exist happily with fungi and microscopic mites in a beneficial ecosystem. Of the larger co-inhabitants of soil, we all know about earthworms that create beautifully aerated and fertilized soil by breaking down grass and leaves and burrowing down into the deeper layers. The smaller organisms such as mites and aphids do the same.

The nature of the soil means that oats can be subject to invasion by fungi. As well as that, aphids (sap-sucking insects) may also carry viruses. This threatens the crop, as do the weeds that will grow in good soil. What happens when chemicals are sprayed onto the oats to get rid of the fungi and the aphids? And what about the weedkillers (herbicides) that the farmer sprays? These pesticides and herbicides provide a result for the farmer: the soil doesn't grow weeds and the oats are free of pests. But what do these chemicals do to the delicate ecosystem of the soil? Rachel Carson explains that the chemicals that indiscriminately sterilise our soils can stay in the soil for many years after the initial spraying episode – even decades. This might explain why even some organic crops continue to contain residues of pesticides. We buy 'organic' vegetables and fruit thinking that they haven't been sprayed with chemicals, but what if this 'organic' produce has been grown on soil that was sterilised a decade earlier?

When oat growers use chemicals that help to protect their crop it has a knock-on effect on the soil. Over time, soil quality is reduced and the crops take up the harmful chemicals as they grow.

What about when the oats are ready for harvest? Once they have grown, they must be harvested in a timely manner so as to not spoil i.e. grow mould. They are then left in storage facilities, often on the farm, until further processing takes place at the packaging plant. During this storage time, the oats can again be subject to contamination – again, mainly from fungi (mould). There is a medical condition called 'Farmer's lung' that causes asthma-like symptoms due to the inhalation of dust-containing moulds. Many of these fungi produce toxins called mycotoxins and, although processing techniques will get rid of the actual fungus, the mycotoxins will remain in the oats. These mycotoxins are detrimental to our health – just as mycotoxins in the mouldy peanuts killed the turkeys I mentioned earlier.

So when we eat our morning oats – a good, healthy breakfast full of fibre and beta-glucan – we must consider what harmful, alien molecules they might also contain. To do this we must think of the soil the oats were grown in, whether or not the crop got infected with fungus or virus, the storage facilities they were kept in and whether or not more mould grew on them. Then we must think about the packaging. Cereal boxes are often made from recyclable paper, so far so good, but the inner bag is often made from plastic derivatives. These plastics have been shown to either release toxic chemicals into the packaging space or cause a migration of the toxin into the food, due to contact with the food (13). The oilier the food, the more migration of plastic occurs. This means that a mouthful of the 'good', beta-glucan containing oats may also come with pesticides, herbicides, mycotoxins and perhaps some plastic derivative. It is these harmful, alien molecules that the body picks up as they pass through the leaky gut and into our bloodstream. And so, I started to wonder whether it was the presence of these harmful, alien molecules that was responsible for hampering the improvement in my oat-eating patients.

Of course, my example centres around oats because this is where I started to look. But I could have just as easily have looked into any cereal or grain that is grown, dried, stored, processed and packaged in this way. Initially I suggested to my patients that they should eliminate gluten and milk from their diet because, in the presence of a leaky gut, gluten and milk can behave like the harmful aliens and pass through the permeable gut into our body. Initially, I thought that gluten and milk were the only uninvited guests to consider. But the oats research opened my eyes to a whole new world of gate crashers. It made me realise that many of the foods that we traditionally think of as being 'good' for us may actually now be 'bad' for us. This is why I tend to put 'good' and 'bad' in quotation marks when referring to food. My patients all want to know what's on the 'good' list and what's on the 'bad' list when it comes to their diet. But after my oats explanation, you'll now be able to see why it can be a bit more complicated than that. It is important not just to understand about the nutrient qualities of our food, but also their likely contaminants.

So which foods can be 'bad' for us even though they appear 'good'? In other words, which foods are more susceptible to toxins? For the Diet to Detox programme I created a list of 'culprit foods' that can contain the harmful, alien, gate crashers of our health – even though there might be nothing wrong with the foods themselves.

GRAINS, NUTS AND PULSES

All cereals and grains that may have been grown, dried and stored like the oats can be subject to mould and chemicals, so these go on the list. Besides oats, that includes wheat, barley, rye, rice and quinoa. Think also of other foods that need to spend long periods of time in storage facilities, either on the farm or in factories, such as pulses like beans, peas, nuts and lentils. These go on the list. But we can also extend this to include any milks that are made from these foods, including nut milks like almond milk, soya milk and any milk made from a grain, cereal or seed.

Another food that you might not quickly associate with dried cereals and grains is beer. This has to go on the list for the same reason as the foods mentioned above. Chocolate also goes on the list, as well as coffee and dried herbs and spices, as they will likely all have been stored and subject to mycotoxins.

FRUIT

Next, let's think of food that happily grows moulds on its surface, like sweet fruits. Remember that much of the fruit we now eat has been bred to provide us with the sweetest hit to our taste buds. I remember growing up as a child in Derbyshire, where apples that came from an orchard would be very tart and sour. Acidic fruits tend to deter the growth of mould on the surface. But most of the fruit we consume is sweet and so all but the acidic fruits – lemon and limes – go on the list of culprit foods.

SUGAR

It is important to note that sweet fruit and sweet food in general, with the exception of blackstrap molasses (or black treacle depending on where you live), also has a negative effect on our gut microbes. I've already mentioned that the gut can be referred to as part of the body's terrain. Let me take this analogy a step further. Imagine that the microbial profiles are trees. The beneficial microbial profile can be seen as the 'good' tree and the harmful microbial profile can be seen as the 'bad' tree. Now, both 'good' and 'bad' trees use sugar as fuel to make them grow. So, if you have good gut health with no gut dysbiosis, you will have more of the 'good' trees than 'bad' trees growing in your gut. If you eat sweet fruit or sweet food, you are mainly feeding the 'good' trees because you don't have so many of the 'bad' trees. This doesn't mean that the 'bad' trees don't grow. It just means that the 'good' trees grow more than the 'bad' trees. Remember it is the 'bad' trees that lead to the production of harmful, alien molecules that damage the gut lining cells. The beneficial molecules that are produced by the 'good' trees, such as butyrate, build and protect the gut lining cells. So, if you don't have gut dysbiosis, eating sweet things may not do too much harm to your gut. However, if you already have gut dysbiosis, eating sweet things is likely to make it worse. So, sweet fruit and sweet foods in general go on the 'culprit foods' list. Wine goes on the list because mould may grow on the surface of the grapes. Pesticides may also have been sprayed on non-organic grapes.

MILK

Animal milk molecules, whether that be proteins and/or sugars, may pass through the leaky gut to trigger the immune system into inflammation. Not only that, when we think of what the animal ate, we are led back to grains. Animals like cows, sheep and goats normally eat grass – they don't normally eat grain. But we humans give them grain to fatten them up. It's interesting that farmers realise this is how to make an animal obese, but we haven't realised this yet for ourselves. If the grain that the animal eats has suffered the same treatment as the grains we eat then it will contain the chemicals and mould toxins we looked at above. In fact, the grain meant for animal consumption may be in a poorer state than that processed for human consumption. This is why it is always best to eat grass-fed meat. Grass eating (ruminant) animals produce a type of fat called conjugated linoleic acid or CLA which has amazing anti-inflammatory and tumour-preventative properties. The sad thing is, when the animal is fed grain, it stops producing CLA. But this isn't the only reason to eat grass-fed meat. Another reason is that if the animal has been fed grain, the mould toxins and chemicals will be in their meat as well as their milk and it will be passed along the food chain to you.

I remember yellow, corn-fed chicken in supermarkets and how this was supposed to be superior to other chicken. The chicken was said to have been fed with omega 3-rich grains. Sadly, I believe this was just a marketing tool. Chickens are omnivores – they eat meat (worms) as well as plant matter.

Fat animals that have been fed grains may well have gut dysbiosis and inflammation. When we eat meat from grain-fed animals we may also be partaking of their inflammation-provoking molecules.

So, the culprit food list can be summed up as follows:

Cereals, grains, including wheat, barley, rye, oats,
    quinoa, rice, pasta
Beans and lentils including chocolate and coffee
Milk including animal, grain and nut milks
Sweet fruit, sweet, processed foods
Alcohol

You might be thinking, "That seems like a lot!" And it is. Am I seriously saying that we should never eat any of these foods ever again? You'll be glad to hear that the answer is no. In the Diet to Detox programme we identify these foods as 'culprit foods' so we know which foods to eliminate *temporarily* in order to heal the gut.

But what happens when we reintroduce these foods into the diet? Aren't we just bringing back all the toxins? Correct. But the beauty of the Diet to Detox programme is that we remove the 'culprit foods' initially so that those holes in the gut lining get a chance to heal. We then start to strengthen the gut by providing it with great microbes. Having healthy microbes also means that the detoxification process also works a lot better. Our gut microbes, working closely with the liver, help us to bio-transform the harmful aliens into molecules that can easily be excreted – either in the faeces, kidneys or through the breath or skin. Once the gut barrier is strong and our detoxification processes are working well, the body should be able to cope with the re-introduction of *some* of the foods on the 'culprit food' list. Of course, you will be much wiser about the origins of your food and so hopefully there will be fewer harmful aliens in the re-introduced foods.

WATER

We've talked about toxins in food, toxins on our skin and toxins in the air. What about toxins in the water we drink? We like to assume that when we turn on the tap to help ourselves to a glass of water, the clear liquid is free from all pollutants. Sadly, this is not the case. One study that looked at global samples of drinking water, found that most of our water contains plastic fibres which can be as big as 0.5 cm. Yep. Half a centimetre. (14). Plastic fibres were also found in 12 samples of beer and 12 samples of sea water (14).

It's perhaps shocking to know that, as well as plastics, pharmaceuticals from hospitals and pharmacies get washed into our water and don't all get removed at the water treatment plants. Research papers show we could be unknowingly medicating ourselves with the water we drink from our kitchen sinks. Painkillers such as ibuprofen and codeine can be present, as well as others such as antibiotics, blood pressure medication, anti-epileptic drugs, anti-depressants and oestrogens.

Water treatment plants do their utmost to ensure that the water that comes out of our taps at home is as safe as they can keep it. However, their own reports admit that they do sometimes experience safety 'failures'. These failures mean that on rare occasions local drinking water can become contaminated with microbes that can harm us, such as *E. Coli,* enterococci, *Clostridium perfringens* and parasites such as cryptosporidium. All of these microbes can cause harm, particularly in those with a compromised immune system such as the very young, the very old and those who are already sick. Heavy metals, including aluminium, iron, and lead can also be found as contamination 'failures' in our drinking water.

These 'failures' thankfully do not happen very often but what is more worrying are the pollutants that are not even detected by water treatment facilities. These *micropollutants* are contaminants found in our water that are not readily identified by water treatment plants. The levels of some, such as pesticides, are regulated. However, the levels of others, such as plastics, pharmaceutical and self-care products, are not regulated. By themselves, the individual toxins may not reach sufficient levels to cause harm. However, studies are now beginning to understand that even if one substance does not cause harm, a mixture of substances is likely to have an appreciable effect on the health of certain individuals.

For the most part, our body tries to eliminate toxins by using our gut microbes and working with the liver, to break them down or bio-transform them into less harmful molecules. However, if there are many toxins present or there is a build-up over time, the system can become overwhelmed and fail. It then allows toxins to enter our body where they get deposited in our tissues. Small amounts accumulate over decades. At some point it is likely that the mix of accumulated toxins plus the development of low-grade chronic inflammation overwhelms the detoxification systems and results in ill health.

In my practice in London, I began to notice that a lot of men were developing small breasts. This is a medical condition called gynaecomastia. After seeing the first few of these, I started to investigate further with blood tests as I knew that gynaecomastia is likely to be caused by female hormones and sometimes these are being produced by tumours. The standard blood tests came back normal, which was reassuring, but I still had no explanation for the 'man-boobs'.

I then attended a lecture about environmental chemicals, particularly endocrine-disrupting chemicals or EDCs, and bingo! I learnt that many toxins act on our endocrine system and disrupt normal function. The National Institute for Environmental Health Sciences (NIEHS) in the US has a section on their website that deals with endocrine disruptors (15). They list some common EDCs, including plastic bottles and the linings of metal cans, detergents, flame retardants, foods such as soy milk, self-care items, toys and pesticides. They state that these endocrine mimickers are 'linked with developmental, reproductive, brain, immune, and other problems.' They also inform us that even small amounts of EDCs can be problematic. Could these EDCs be present in our water? Could the EDCs be responsible for the increased incidence of 'man-boobs'? I can't give a definitive answer to these questions but as toxins are everywhere, it is of course likely that the combinations of toxins has an additive effect on our health.

EDCs can affect the development of the growing baby in its mother's womb. The NIEHS pioneered the work into understanding the drug diethylstilbestrol (DES). This drug was given to pregnant women from the 1940s to the 1970s to prevent miscarriage. DES caused epigenetic changes in the baby and resulted in an increased rate of a rare form of vaginal cancer.

As well as cancers, EDCs may cause disordered sexual organ development. A number of studies are now looking at the situation of intersex fish as a result of EDCs that are in our rivers. I previously mentioned that we used to live in the South of France. France is one of the leading countries for science and medical research and I was once chatting to a group of PhD students in Provence. One had recently arrived to start her research in a local research institute. I asked her what she was working on and she told me that she was about to start working under a professor who was researching the subject of the feminisation of male fish due to the effects of oestrogens in the river waters. It may be that oestrogens, or chemicals that mimic oestrogens, in our rivers and our drinking water were the cause of the 'man-boobs' in my patients. We may not hear about it but the research into intersex fish has been underway for some time and indicates just how important EDCs are (16).

It also seems that cocktails of similar acting EDCs will have a far greater effect on the body than individual EDCs (17). For example, pesticides and plastics both mimic oestrogen and block the action of normal oestrogen in our bodies. We are bombarded by these cocktails of chemicals from the air we breathe, the water we drink, the food we eat and even the clothes we wear. What is unclear is how this silent accumulation of toxins in our environment will affect the next generation of children.

NON-PHYSICAL TOXINS

We've talked about the usual suspects of physical toxins – the air we breathe, the water we drink and the food we eat. But what about non-physical toxins? When I help people on their journey to wellbeing, I have found that there are two main areas that can present as a roadblock on this journey. One is toxins from teeth amalgams or root canals or other bodily implants e.g. breast implants. The other is non-physical toxins. Non-physical toxins such as those coming from electromagnetic frequency (EMF) waves or from subconscious, psychological, emotional or spiritual issues can derail your best efforts to re-organise your diet and physical environment.

In chapter 1 we learnt that we are electric beings. Our thoughts can be picked up as electricity on brain tracings called EEGs. Just as a coiled wire that carries an electrical charge will create a magnetic field, in the human body, the DNA helix acts as a coiled string of molecules that carry electricity and hence produce a magnetic field. But what has this to do with non-physical toxins and roadblocks to health? Well, not only do our bodies project an electromagnetic force but our bodies can be *changed* by electromagnetic forces. So electromagnetic fields – for example from electricity cabling and WIFI devices – may have an effect on our body's functioning.

As far as our electromagnetic thoughts are concerned, they too have an effect on our DNA. This isn't conjecture. Studies show that our thoughts can affect the structure and function of our DNA (18). I often find that individuals who are sensitive to their emotional surroundings are also sensitive to WIFI devices. My son Harry was one such individual. I also find that the WIFI-sensitive individuals are also likely to have leaky gut. My son Harry ticked all of these boxes. As a family, we noticed that if Harry spent more than a couple of hours on any device, including watching TV, his mood would take a nosedive. This would be even worse if he had been eating culprit foods. Over the years he has learned to monitor screen time and food. He knows that if his mood is feeling particularly low, he must check what he's eating and cut down on screen time. Harry will also get physical pain in his leg if he keeps his mobile phone in his pocket for extended periods of time.

I've learned over the years that it is best to deal with any subconscious, emotional, psychological or spiritual issues before embarking upon Diet to Detox. It's fascinating how food has the ability to reveal our innermost struggles. When we embark upon the elimination part of the Diet to Detox, this is when the inner turmoil is revealed. People who deal with the mental, emotional, subconscious and spiritual toxins (MESS) first, find that the Diet to Detox programme is a much more enjoyable journey. I use breathing techniques and a muscle testing technique called Neuromodulation Therapy (NMT) to help to resolve any of the hidden issues before suggesting that my patients start on Diet to Detox.

SO WHAT CAN WE DO ABOUT TOXINS?

When we think about the toxins that surround us – in our environment, our food and our self-care items, it's easy to feel despondent. How could we possibly eliminate all those toxins? The answer is: we can't. Many of the toxins in our environment, and even in our food, are more or less unavoidable. There are actions we can take to avoid them, like eating grass-fed meat and choosing toxin-free cosmetics, but it is impossible to avoid all toxins from getting into our bodies. So what can we do about toxins?

As we've seen, most of the usual suspect categories of toxins (heavy metals, moulds, plastics, pesticides) either behave as DNA adducts, cause direct damage to the DNA and the gut, or act as endocrine disruptors. And most patients I measure have more than one toxin in their body. This can seem depressing but I'm happy to tell you that people do get better. The body is a wonderful thing and is designed to get rid of toxins. Through the gut, the skin, sweating and through the urine, we are designed to expel unwanted aliens. The gut, in combination with the liver and gall bladder, helps us to detoxify from harmful molecules, transforming the substance into something less harmful through biotransformation. The body is then able to expel the substance through the easiest possible route. Sweating after exercise or in a sauna is helpful at eliminating many petrol-derived toxins (19). But the easiest way to help our body to get rid of toxins is through the food we eat. Certain foods are vitally important in helping us to detoxify and are the main reason I have written this book.

Populations around the world have eaten fermented foods for centuries. Of course, there are myriad different fermented foods, but there seems to be some recurring themes when it comes to the microbes that are involved in the detoxification or biotransformation process. For example, lactic acid bacteria are a common feature in many fermented foods and studies show that different types of lactic acid bacteria are able to deal with the usual suspect categories of heavy metals, moulds, plastics, and pesticides. After all that doom and gloom, this is good news! It might seem crazy to think that the humble fermented cabbage, which produces strains of lacto-bacilli, will help us to detoxify from dangerous illness-inducing toxins – but it does.

Societies like the Japanese, that eat fermented food regularly, tend to stay well. This is because not only do the fermented foods provide nutrients and microbes, but they also help the body to get rid of the harmful aliens. Introducing fermented food should be a relatively simple thing to do, except for two problems. One is that, in developed countries, we have forgotten what a fermented food is. When I say the word fermentation, most people can only think of cabbage and beer. This book will hopefully change that and introduce a whole new repertoire of dishes for you to enjoy.

The second problem we have when we want to introduce fermented food is that if we already have gut dysbiosis, adding fermented food may actually makes things worse. I'll talk more about this when I introduce the Diet to Detox programme, but for now we just need to understand that, if we are not used to them, we should introduce fermented foods gently so as not to cause an upset in the gut and other systems. But once you've established a regular regime of delicious recipes, you can expect your health to improve as your body is naturally able to get rid of toxins.

1. Poirier MC. Chemical-induced DNA damage and human cancer risk. Discovery medicine. 2012;14:283.
2. Patterson E, Cryan JF, Fitzgerald GF, Ross RP, Dinan TG, Stanton C. Gut microbiota, the pharmabiotics they produce and host health. Proc Nutr Soc. 2014;73:477-489.
3. Lang O. Dietary Adequacy among the native Eskimo. Bachelor's Diploma Dissertation, Masaryk University, Czech Republic, viewed on. 2017;19
4. Wibowo MC, Yang Z, Borry M et al. Reconstruction of ancient microbial genomes from the human gut. Nature. 20211-6.
5. Claesson MJ, Jeffery IB, Conde S et al. Gut microbiota composition correlates with diet and health in the elderly. Nature. 2012;488:178-184.
6. UK CR. What's in a cigarette? Available from: https://www. cancerresearchuk.org/about-cancer/causes-of-cancer/smoking-and-cancer/ whats-in-a-cigarette-0
7. Pauly JL, Paszkiewicz G. Cigarette smoke, bacteria, mold, microbial toxins, and chronic lung inflammation. Journal of oncology. 2011;2011
8. Dominguez A, Fagan JM. Toxins in Cosmetics. 2015
9. Manikkam M, Haque MM, Guerrero-Bosagna C, Nilsson EE, Skinner MK. Pesticide methoxychlor promotes the epigenetic transgenerational inheritance of adult-onset disease through the female germline. PloS one. 2014;9:e102091.
10. Mail D. Toxic levels of air pollution are behind a record spike in asthma deaths: Official figures reveal a 25 per cent jump in a decade prompting calls for urgent action to tackle the crisis. 2021. Available from: https://www. dailymail.co.uk/health/article-5969727/Toxic-levels-air-pollution-record-spike-asthma-deaths.html
11. Luosujärvi RA, Husman TM, Seuri... M. Joint symptoms and diseases associated with moisture damage in a health center. Clinical 2003
12. Carson R. Silent spring. Houghton Mifflin Harcourt; 2002
13. Hahladakis JN, Velis CA, Weber R, Iacovidou E, Purnell P. An overview of chemical additives present in plastics: Migration, release, fate and environmental impact during their use, disposal and recycling. Journal of hazardous materials. 2018;344:179-199.
14. Kosuth M, Mason SA, Wattenberg EV. Anthropogenic contamination of tap water, beer, and sea salt. PloS one. 2018;13:e0194970.
15. Sciences NIOEH. Endocrine disruptors. 2021. Available from: https:// www.niehs.nih.gov/health/topics/agents/endocrine/index.cfm
16. Minier C, Caltot G, Leboulanger F, Hill EM. An investigation of the incidence of intersex fish in Seine-Maritime and Sussex region. Analusis. 2000;28:801-806.
17. Kortenkamp A. Ten years of mixing cocktails: a review of combination effects of endocrine-disrupting chemicals. Environmental health perspectives. 2007
18. McCraty R, Atkinson M, Tomasino D. Modulation of DNA conformation by heart-focused intention. ... Center. 2003
19. Schnare DW, Ben M, Shields MG. Body burden reductions of PCBs, PBBs and chlorinated pesticides in human subjects. Ambio. 1984

CHAPTER 5

THE DIET TO DETOX

Diet to Detox is based around my view that toxins are, more often than not, the underlying trigger for ill health. As we've seen, toxins can have a direct effect on our DNA or on body tissues and they can also damage the gut microbiota, causing gut dysbiosis or 'leaky gut'. The gut is said to be an immune organ in its own right, rather like the spleen. The more research work that is done to look at the gut, the more we find this to be true. This means that toxins, in harming the gut, harm our immune system.

The cells of the immune system, the Ninja peas, are the main guardians of our health. They look out for infections that gain access to our body through the leaky gut and destroy them. They also look out for other harmful 'alien' molecules that might cause hay fever or an allergy and deal with those. And they look out for cells that have gone rogue and want to turn into cancer cells and they deal with these too. If our Ninja cells are well, we are well. If our Ninja cells are sick, we are sick.

When we have gut dysbiosis, the passage of harmful aliens through the porous gut means that the Ninja peas are always working. This creates a chronic and often silent inflammation that uses up the body's resources of vitamins, minerals and hormones. At this stage we may begin to notice some symptoms of fatigue or a feeling of being 'run down'. We might get a blood test done and find that some vitamin levels are low. We might see a functional medicine doctor, naturopath or nutritional therapist who might also diagnose adrenal fatigue. Correcting the imbalance in vitamins, minerals or hormones may help us to return to health.

If left unchecked, the chronic silent inflammation may eventually form DNA adducts and alter DNA function, causing the epigenetic 'switch' to flip. This is when our symptoms become more significant and we are diagnosed with a specific condition. When we stand back and examine this process from afar, we can see the Hierarchy of Health at play. The 'diagnosis' is really a symptom of the toxins damaging the cells and damaging the gut. Whereas mainstream medicine would choose to deal with the diagnosis, Diet to Detox deals with the cause – which is the toxins. So, the three main areas of concern in the Hierarchy of Health (and therefore in Diet to Detox) are:

1 *Toxins*
2 *The gut*
3 *The immune cells*

The three phases of Diet to Detox aim to:

1 *Remove the toxins*
2 *Heal the gut*
3 *Heal the Ninja peas*

When we remove the toxins from our environment, we allow the cells to recover and resume normal function. Removing toxins is the first step to healing the gut. The second step is to give the gut lining cells and our own resident microbes the right food and environment in which to flourish. This usually means giving the gut nutrient-dense, non-toxic foods that feed the large intestine.

The immune cells are ever vigilant. However, like all other cells, they need to regenerate themselves. Have you ever considered why it is that we just sometimes need a break, that holiday in the sun, when we don't do much other than read a good book, soak up the vitamin D and sleep? When we down tools from a busy or stressful life, we allow our body to recover so that we feel refreshed and ready to go back to our busy and stressful life (there must be a wider message in that sentence).

Like our body as a whole, the Ninja immune cells need time off to recover. To prevent the silent inflammation from becoming a diagnosis, we must give the Ninja peas a holiday. By allowing the gut to heal, we are also giving the Ninja cells a rest from their combat activities. If the gut isn't letting harmful aliens through the gaps in the gut border wall then the Ninja peas have less work to do. Once the leaky gut is no longer leaky, the immune cells are able to regenerate themselves. Again, eating nutrient-dense, non-toxic foods will allow the Ninja cells to recover and be ready to resume service.

When we achieve the three main aims of Diet to Detox, inflammation is reduced. Lower levels of inflammation mean that the body uses fewer resources, which means that our vitamin, mineral and hormone levels are maintained. Having a system replete of these resources means that we are less likely to develop chronic disease. Let me put that the other way round.

We are less likely to develop chronic disease if we have

- *fewer toxins*
- *a good gut barrier*
- *reduced inflammation*
- *good vitamin, mineral and hormone levels*

Diet to Detox is designed to help you to achieve this. Let's look at an overview of how it works before we delve into each phase in more detail.

PHASE I DIET TO DETOX
In Phase I of Diet to Detox, we temporarily eliminate the culprit toxic foods. The aim here is to

- *Allow the gut microbes to recover a normal gut profile*
- *Allow the Ninja peas to forget their sensitivity to toxins*
- *Stop allowing DNA adduct formation*
- *Stop any other direct damage to cells*

Please note that a true food allergy such as an allergy to nuts, where there is an immediate anaphylactic reaction or a reaction requiring an Epipen, does not respond to Diet to Detox.

Gut dysbiosis is linked to food sensitivity reactions rather than true allergies. Gut dysbiosis allows the passage of harmful 'alien' molecules or toxins which would not normally gain entrance into the body. As it is the toxins that cause the gut dysbiosis, the first step is to remove the toxins. As I've mentioned previously, the food itself, such as whole grains, may be 'good' for your health. However, the toxin that it comes with, will still cause you harm. The Ninja immune cells are very clever. Once they have seen a toxin they will remember that toxin for quite a while. Then, when faced with the toxin again, they can instantly react. This reaction might be in the form of causing a stomach upset, pain in the abdomen or worsening of joint and muscle pain, brain fog or fatigue. These are called food sensitivity or hypersensitivity reactions. It's great that the Ninja pea recognises the toxin. However, what it also does is recognise the food that is associated with the toxin. For example, if the mould toxin comes with a grain, the Ninja peas will remember the grain-mould combination. In other words, the Ninja peas remembers the whole food-toxin complex, not just the toxin. They seem to be able to take a copy of the whole food-toxin complex and remember every little part of it. This means that after the Ninja peas have become sensitised to the food-toxin complex, if they then meet the food – even if it is not with the toxin – it will react to the food as if it were the whole food-toxin complex. This creates inflammation every time that food is eaten, even if it is not with the toxin. The subsequent inflammation and Ninja exhaustion will ultimately make the gut dysbiosis worse. This means that more and more foods get added to the list of foods the person can't eat. And this is why you need to give your Ninja cells a break from meeting up with the food-toxin complex. By giving the Ninja peas a complete break from this relationship, they are able to 'forget' that they know the food-toxin complex. Then when you reintroduce the food later on, the good food no longer triggers an inflammatory cascade.

Of course, I am oversimplifying these very complex mechanisms, whereas immunologists write whole books on just this topic. I probably could not explain in immunological terms what I have experienced to be true in real life. What I see in real life is that if you remove the culprit foods for a period of time – that is, usually in the region of six weeks – the person can often then reintroduce the food and not see any symptoms. I must re-state however, that this is not the situation for someone who has a true allergy to a food.

But isn't this just like any other elimination diet? Not quite. One example of an elimination diet is the FODMAP diet. The FODMAP diet was developed by Monash University in Australia and is often recommended for people suffering from irritable bowel syndrome (IBS). Short chain fermentable sugars in foods such as wheat, milk, mushrooms, onions and nuts, to name a few, are avoided. The FODMAP diet has helped a great many people. However, what I increasingly see is that the person feels great for a while whilst avoiding the prescribed foods, but then at some point they begin to react to more and more foods. My son Luke was like this. Initially, he felt fine when he avoided gluten and milk but then as time progressed, we realised that he started to have seemingly random reactions to other foods. One day he came home and we realised that he was now intolerant to paprika, as this had been the only new ingredient in a take-away meal that he had eaten.

What I understand to be happening here is that, although the main food-toxin complexes are being avoided, toxins associated with other foods are still being taken in and are causing inflammation as they do so. With the paprika, this spice is likely to have been dried and therefore may have been associated with mould during processing or storage. Elimination diets like FODMAP or diets where nightshades or histamine-provoking foods are avoided, for example, fail to take the toxins into consideration. It's the toxin that harms the gut microbial profile and creates inflammation when nightshades are eaten or creates more histamine than it should with other foods. When we remove the toxin, we allow restoration of normal function to both the gut, the gut microbial profile, the inflammation levels *and* the immune cells. Many of my patients tell me that after following Diet to Detox they can re-introduce foods that they were previously sensitive to.

PHASE II DIET TO DETOX

If Phase I Diet to Detox is about giving the gut and the immune cells a rest, Phase II Diet to Detox is about repairing the broken wall and shoring up the gut defences. This process will have already begun in Phase I. Removing the toxins will allow a return to normal for the gut microbiota. Eating food that nourishes the colon will also help to repair the gut barrier wall. In Phase II Diet to Detox, we take the repair process to the next level. How do we do this? By introducing fermented foods. When I first start talking about fermented food with my patients, they often don't really know what I mean. Fermented food, to the uninitiated, often means sauerkraut. But there is so much more to fermented food than that and hopefully by the time you have finished this book and tried the recipes, you'll be hooked forever.

But what exactly *are* fermented foods? Let's look first at the traditions we have in the western world surrounding fermented foods. Beer and wine are easy ones. These are made from fermented grains and fermented grapes. The ferment used to make beer and wine is called *Saccharomyces cerevisiae*. Although fermentation is used in the production process, the increase in alcohol that occurs during this process kills off the yeast, so that there is none left in the final drink.

Bread is another food that uses the fermentation process. *Saccharomyces cerevisiae,* used as brewer's yeast in beer and wine making, is the same yeast – sometimes called baker's yeast – used in bread making. The yeast digests the grains and releases carbon dioxide and alcohol, just like in the beer and wine making process. It's the bubbles from the carbon dioxide and the alcohol that make the bread rise. When baked in the oven most of the yeast (and other microbes that form during the proofing) dies, and the alcohol burns off.

So what about traditional foods eaten in the western world that have live microbes when we consume them? We have, of course, milk products like yoghurts and cheeses. We are familiar with these fermented foods although, sadly, many that are available in our supermarkets no longer contain live microbes. Less well known are cured meats, like bacon, pastrami, chorizo and salami (1). These are salted and left to dry for anything from a few days to a few years. During this process, the meat becomes colonised by beneficial microbes which ferment it, leaving beneficial molecules and wonderful flavours. Another fermented or probiotic food that you may not be aware of is olives in brine. Olives stored in salt water will grow beneficial microbes on their surface. Of course, you will also be consuming good anti-inflammatory molecules along with the probiotics. Having a few olives with your meal is an easy way to add a fermented food to your diet.

So, in Phase II of Diet to Detox, we begin to add fermented foods. At first, we still avoid the culprit foods, even if they are fermented, although there is room for rule-bending depending on how you are responding. I've already mentioned sauerkraut, which is perhaps the most well-known fermented food. Sauerkraut is a traditional eastern European dish and is quite acidic for some people's palates. However, sauerkraut isn't the only fermented cabbage in town. I will introduce you to many different ways of fermenting cabbage and I'm sure you will find one that suits you. Cabbage is one of the cheapest and easiest ways to introduce fermented food and it comes with so many health benefits. Not only do you get a healthy dose of probiotic microbes, you also get a wide array of vitamins and anti-inflammatory molecules. I will also introduce you to other fermented vegetables and I'll be showing you just how simple they are to make. Once you start to ferment vegetables and see how delicious they become, you'll never go back to the old ways. You will also be introduced to fermented proteins such as fermented salmon mousse and fermented hummus. Phase II Diet to Detox is fun, and you'll discover a whole new realm of food, cooking and eating.

If fermented foods are so good for us, why don't we start adding them at the beginning of Diet to Detox? When I first discovered the importance of the gut, I used to tell my patients to eat plenty of fermented foods. However, I soon realised that this wasn't the best way to start. As already mentioned, the most commonly known fermented food, sauerkraut, is quite acidic. Many people found that eating sauerkraut aggravated any stomach acidity or indigestion that they had. Other people found that eating fermented foods made them ill. Some people would even be made ill by taking probiotics. Why was this? I briefly mentioned earlier a condition called Small Intestinal Bacterial Overgrowth or SIBO. This is when there are too many microbes living in the upper gut. Under normal circumstances, there are very few microbes living in the upper intestine, as most live in the colon. When there are too many growing in the upper gut, they tend to take food that arrives there and start to ferment it immediately. This process is normally done lower down in the large intestine. When fermentation happens in the upper gut, gas is produced and the result is bloating and wind after eating. Eating probiotic foods can aggravate the situation still further in that the microbes in the food interact with the microbes in the upper gut. This reaction may result in indigestion, diarrhoea, constipation and fatigue.

Another problem with introducing fermented foods too early is the presence of gut dysbiosis. The permeable, 'leaky' gut may allow passage of the probiotic microbes into the body. Again, under normal circumstances, the probiotic microbes should stay in the gut because the gap junctions that exist between the gut lining cells prevent microbes from entering into the body. But even 'good' probiotic microbes can cause a systemic infection or inflammation in the body if not dealt with adequately by the Ninja immune cells. I will talk more about this later. The combination of reactions I've just described may lead to many unwanted symptoms. This is why we must first fix the holes in the gut and encourage the growth of our own beneficial gut microbes in the large intestine before we introduce fermented foods.

When we do introduce fermented foods, we take a slow and steady approach. When I started with my kids, I made a fair few mistakes when introducing fermented foods. Take kombucha. Kombucha is fermented green tea and, made well, it can be crisp and light. It goes down really well – so well in fact that you could be forgiven for thinking that it is a harmless fizzy drink. How wrong you would be! This deliciously refreshing drink is packed with probiotic microbes. This makes it very powerful. When I first gave some to my son Luke, he had been suffering from gut dysbiosis for a while. He didn't have very many gut symptoms apart from bad breath, but he was easily fatigued and couldn't manage a full session of swim training without having to sleep for several hours afterwards. I gave him just 5mls of kombucha – yes, just one teaspoon – and he reacted with fatigue, bloating and diarrhoea and felt unwell for a number of days. I waited a few weeks before trying again with half a teaspoon, and this time he was fine. We then gradually increased the amount until he could freely drink a full glass of kombucha. As it is so delicious, he would then happily drink half a bottle at a time (he's a big guy). Kombucha can be expensive, so it was at this point that I started to make my own. You'll find an easy kombucha recipe in the recipe section.

PHASE III DIET TO DETOX

In Phase III Diet to Detox, we reintroduce the foods we eliminated in Phase I. It is important that we are already eating a variety of fermented foods, introduced in Phase II, before we begin this phase. The fermented foods shore up the gut defences so that, if we should add a food that the gut or immune system does not like, we can cope with the after effects without becoming too unwell. The aim here is to reintroduce a culprit food to see if the immune system still does not like it. As mentioned earlier, the immune system may not like a particular food because it associates the food with a toxin. Another reason for not liking a food is because of a true allergy or because of an inability to digest the food because of a missing enzyme. Most people know when they have a true allergy to a food. They might have been diagnosed with this allergy from childhood and may have a specific reaction such as swelling of the mouth, wheezing or difficulty breathing and/or abdominal pain. They may need to use an Epipen to immediately reduce the hypersensitivity reaction. If you have a true allergy or know that you have never been able to eat a certain food, please do continue to stay away from these foods.

It is also important to know when your gut is ready to accept the challenge of the old foods. How do we know that the gut is ready? This, for me, has a relatively simple and straight forward answer: We know the gut has healed when there are no symptoms and you are passing three soft stools per day. If you no longer have your previous symptoms, this is likely to mean that inflammation levels have gone down, which in turn means that the gut and immune system are functioning well. Further evidence of the gut functioning well is the bowels being open three times per day with soft stools, no pain and no bloating. If this has been happening for two weeks, then you're ready for Phase III.

When reintroducing foods, again you need to be patient. Slow and steady wins the day. You may by this stage be feeling great, with improved energy levels and no gut symptoms. People may start to comment about how well you look and your skin may be glowing. It can be tempting to think you are now totally healed and can dive back into the old stuff. This is where the maximum restraint is needed. I find that if patients go too fast at this stage, it can be difficult to re-establish the rhythm. In fact, it can take several weeks to return to wellbeing once you fall off the wagon. So, take one food at a time. Choose a food that you didn't have a reaction to previously. For example, if you used to have bloating and fatigue after eating dairy or gluten, leave these food groups to the end.

Another way to make the transition smoother is to choose a 'culprit food' that can be fermented. For example, you may already be enjoying fermented coconut milk. You could now add pureed fruit to the coconut milk and leave it to sit (covered) on the countertop overnight before enjoying the next day. This way you are using the probiotic microbes in the coconut milk to start pre-digesting the fruit sugars and break down any toxins in the fruit. It is a good idea to do this with as many of the culprit foods as you can before you introduce a completely non-fermented culprit food. You can even add my own special Ferment Blend (see website store) to coffee powder and let it sit overnight before brewing your coffee. Of course, you could then make a fermented ice coffee! For chocolate, look for some of my fermented chocolate recipes. You'll find that there are a lot of Phase III ferments that incorporate culprit foods, so don't worry, those old friends will be back.

Remember, slow and steady is the order of the day. Introduce one food per week and don't overdo that one food. For example, if it's fermented chocolate mousse, on the first day have one teaspoon. If the next day you are still feeling great, have two teaspoons, and if the next day after that there are still no negative reactions, try a dessert spoon. If the day after that, you're still OK, try two dessert spoons and continue in this same fashion as you go through the week. The next week, you can then try adding another food. Start again with one teaspoon of that new food and double the quantity each day if you have no negative reactions.

What happens if you have a reaction to a food? If you have a reaction such as bloating, indigestion, fatigue, joint pains or a return of previous symptoms, stop the culprit food and don't add any further foods until your symptoms have settled down. Wait at least five days after your symptoms have settled before you try a different food. The food that caused the symptoms should be relegated to the bottom of the challenge list to be re-tried at a later date.

Now that we can see how the three phases of Diet to Detox work, we can look at each phase in more detail. So first, let's deal with those culprit foods.

CHAPTER 6

PHASE I DIET TO DETOX ELIMINATING TOXINS

In Phase I of Diet to Detox, we eliminate the culprit toxic foods. The aim here is to

- *Allow the gut microbes to recover a normal gut profile*
- *Allow the Ninja peas/immune system to forget their sensitivity to toxins*
- *Stop allowing DNA adduct formation*
- *Stop any other direct damage to cells from toxins*

Once we accomplish these goals, many illnesses and conditions will be greatly improved. The list of culprit foods is given below:

CATEGORY	EXAMPLE	EXCEPTIONS OR SUBSTITUTE
GRAINS, CEREALS	*Wheat, barley, rye, oats, quinoa, rice, pasta. Oat or grain milks.*	*Konjac noodles, Kanten noodles, edamame noodles*
ANIMAL MILK	*All animal milks, yoghurt, cheese, kefir.*	*Coconut milk*
SUGARS	*Refined sugars e.g. cakes and biscuits, all fruit juice, all fruit*	*Lemons, limes Molasses*
NUTS	*All nuts, almonds, soya beans. All nut milks including soya and almond milks.*	
BEANS, PEAS, LENTILS	*Including canned beans and lentils. All bean milks.*	*Fresh or frozen garden peas, or green beans, edamame beans*
SEEDS, SPICES	*All seeds and spices*	*Freshly grown herbs*
CHOCOLATE	*All chocolate*	
COFFEE	*All coffee*	
ALCOHOL	*All alcohol*	

Visit www.doctorese.com

For some people, this list can make pretty grim reading. In my clinics, when patients come to me with painful joints and/or gut-related inflammation symptoms, I can often predict what they eat for breakfast. It's usually oats or cereal of some description, perhaps muesli with milk or yoghurt. There may also be some nuts and/or seeds and berries thrown on top. All in all, you'd say that this was a pretty healthy breakfast. But of course, if you've read the preceding chapters, you'll know that this description of breakfast includes a good proportion of the culprit foods. In fact, breakfast is often the main 'culprit meal'. Do you remember why? Because the grains and cereals (the definition of what makes a grain and what makes a cereal is not important) can grow moulds whilst growing in the fields and whilst sitting in storage. During food processing, manufacturers will try to get rid of the mould from the outsides of the plant but will not succeed in getting rid of the mould toxins, or mycotoxins, that invade inside the plant. When you eat cereals and grains regularly, whether or not they taste or smell of mould, you may be consuming some degree of mycotoxin.

Moulds and mycotoxins are not the only thing that can be ingested with the cereals or grains. Unless explicitly indicated, the plant is likely to have been sprayed to prevent insect infestation. This means your morning cereal will also provide you with a dose of at least two toxins. And remember that the packaging is also important, as plastic can leach into the food. This adds another toxin to make at least three. Of course, if you drink water from the tap you are likely to increase this number greatly. Eating a good healthy breakfast of cereals, nuts, seeds, fruit and yoghurt may be inextricably combined with toxins. Thus, many people who think they are eating healthily are inadvertently making themselves ill.

A WORD ABOUT BEER AND WINE

Even though there is no ferment left in the final drink, this isn't to say that beer and wine are not good for the colon. Did I say that? Yes! When the yeast ferments the grain or the wine, they create wonderful bioactive substances. Guinness beer made in Ireland is known to be rich in B vitamins. A Spanish study found that moderate beer drinking could provide Vitamins B2, B3, B6, B12 and folate (2). Most people also know that red wine has been shown to be beneficial for health. Studies are clear that moderate consumption of red wine results in a reduction in heart attacks, strokes, diabetes and cholesterol (3). Moderate beer drinking has also been shown to increase HDL, the good cholesterol (3). Also, moderate consumption of both beer and red wine are associated with a lowered risk of cancer (3). One study found that drinking one unit of beer per day (about 220mls of 5.5 % ABV beer) reduced the risk of prostate cancer (3). Of course, if you drink too much alcohol, the body produces too many harmful free radicals which harm the liver and cause inflammation. Regular, moderate consumption, rather than binge drinking, is the key. Most government authorities in the UK and US would suggest one drink (150 ml of wine or 10g of alcohol) daily for women and two drinks (300 ml of wine or 20g of alcohol) daily for men.

It's great to know that there is good to be had from drinking in moderation. However – and here comes the negative part – very few research papers mention the toxins and the negative effect on health from consuming these toxins with your beer or wine. If you drank one or two glasses per day of mycotoxin- or pesticide-enhanced beer or wine, this certainly would not be good for your health. This is why you must avoid alcohol in Phase I.

So how long must we avoid the culprit foods in Phase I Diet to Detox? For most people, this is going to be in the region of six weeks. However, this time frame is sometimes shorter. A patient of mine called Ron was due to have a hip replacement. He was in his early fifties and came to me to see if there was anything he could do to prolong the time before he would need the operation. We talked about culprit foods and, sure enough, the culprit breakfast was a prominent meal in Ron's life. I explained to him about Diet to Detox and he was keen to give it go. I also explained the link between inflammation and pain. Ron had a diagnosis of severe osteoarthritis of the hips. This means that he had severe 'wear and tear' of the hip ball and socket joints. In practice, this usually reveals itself as painful restricted hip movements. I examined Ron and this is exactly what he had. He could barely internally rotate his hips and movement was painful. I explained to Ron that it was the inflammation that caused the pain and not the wear and tear. It is perhaps counter-intuitive to say this because often we think that the worn-out ball and socket must be rubbing against each other and that this is the cause of the pain. But during my sport and exercise medicine training, we were taught that we must not 'treat the MRI'. What do I mean by this? For a patient with severe osteoarthritis, the X-Ray or MRI images will look pretty depressing. The bones are gnarly and the cartilage is eaten away so that there may appear to be no space in the joint. The surgeons often use the term 'bone on bone' for this appearance. However, if you ask the patient if they are in constant pain due to this 'bone on bone' grinding, they will often say 'no'. Often the pain will come and go. If the ball was truly scraping the socket with each movement, surely each step would be agony? In fact, what I've found is that, if you treat the inflammation, the pain is greatly improved. This is because pain is linked to inflammation. Research literature backs this up but in mainstream medicine we still insist on treating the MRI.

Ron gave Diet to Detox a try and within two weeks his pain was gone. I explained to him that he was still likely to have a degree of stiffness as the anatomy of the joint would not change, but the inflammation would greatly improve. In just two weeks Ron could now contemplate the fact that he might not need the operation after all. It's important to note that, if I had given Ron another MRI at this point, the images would not have changed. His joints would still look gnarly and have that 'bone on bone' appearance. What changed was the inflammation and, with it, Ron's pain. You might be as fortunate as Ron and have a rapid response. Children also often respond very quickly like this too, sometimes within days. However, the majority of people will need around six weeks to respond to Phase I Diet to Detox – and of course, not everyone responds at all.

ROADBLOCKS: WHO DOESN'T RESPOND TO DIET TO DETOX?
The people who tend not to respond to Diet to Detox are often those with an internal source of physical toxins such as

- *Dental fillings*
- *Root canal treatment*
- *Implants e.g. teeth, breast, joint replacements*

I often advise patients to see a holistic dentist if they have a lot of old metal fillings or have had root canal treatments. A good holistic dentist will be able to tell the patient if the fillings and root canals are a source of toxins. The toxins can be from metals such as mercury and others as described previously, but they can also be from chronic low-grade infection in the jaw. These low-grade infections or cavitations can be a constant source of toxic material leaching from the jaw and keeping the immune system busy. It is, for the most part, a silent process. For many decades, the patient will have no symptoms at all. There may eventually be some low-level pain associated with a tooth or the jaw. This may be identified as an abscess by a conventional dentist, however, the dentist may still not appreciate that there is an underlying 'bed' of infection that has given rise to the abscess. If there is no presentation like an abscess, the holistic dentist will need to do specific imaging to identify cavitations or chronic jaw infection.

In my experience these chronic infections in the jaw can be quite marked and extensive. Following the Diet to Detox plan can greatly help to control the levels of inflammation that result from this chronic infectious process, but ultimately some level of intervention from the holistic dentist will be needed. I get the impression that dental toxins as a source of insult to the DNA and the gut are much more common that we think.

Of course, as I mentioned previously, toxins are not always physical in nature. Dealing with your MESS (mental, emotional, subconscious and spiritual issues) is as important as dealing with your physical toxins. I mentioned that I use a form of therapy called NeuroModulation Therapy (NMT) to help patients to access MESS issues. In fact, NMT deals with both physical and non-physical aspects of health but I find it indispensable to access the areas that prevent progress in my Diet to Detox programme. Interestingly, there is also evidence that using NMT can reduce the level of dental cavitations (4).

There is another category of people who tend not to respond to Diet to Detox and this is people taking immunosuppressive medication for autoimmune types of inflammation such as rheumatoid arthritis (RA). Most of the modern-day medications prescribed for RA suppress the immune system. These types of medications revolutionized the treatment of RA and many people are helped by them. However, for a lot of people, the medication will work for a time and then side effects may dictate a change to another immunosuppressant. I never recommend that patients come off medications prescribed by their rheumatologist. However, when we work to enhance gut and immune health, we are, in effect, trying to 'wake up' or re-establish proper function of the immune system. This cannot happen if the immune system is already controlled by the medications. The problem is, stopping medications abruptly can result in an unpleasant flare-up of disease. In order to re-establish a proper gut–immune system function we need to be able to come off medication without flaring up the disease. This requires close liaison between the patient, their rheumatologist and myself. Few rheumatologists understand what I do so, sadly, I hardly ever get to work to re-establish wellbeing in such patients.

If there are no 'roadblocks' you will see some gentle signs of recovery within the first few weeks. For example, your mood may change reasonably quickly. As we saw in chapter 1, serotonin is formed in the gut. Once the gut starts to recover, I often see the mood lift. Brain fog may also start to improve. Again, low serotonin levels may contribute to brain fog and so the patient may see some improvement in this area early in Diet to Detox. Constipation can sometimes also be improved early in Phase I. However, this is highly variable and constipation can sometimes get worse for a period of time. Constipation is a huge topic all of its own and it is sometimes associated with MESS issues (if you excuse my pun). If you would like to understand more about this issue, refer to the constipation module on my website *www.doctorese.com*.

'WAVY' REACTIONS

Progress with the Diet to Detox programme is almost never linear. What I mean by this is that, unlike when you take a medicine, you may not feel better and better each day. Your progress may follow a wavy curve, with symptoms sometimes getting better and sometimes getting worse, and so moving in a wave-like, up-and-down fashion. However, the overall trend is upwards to recovery.

I believe this wavy reaction occurs for three reasons. The first possible explanation is known as the 'Jarisch-Herxheimer' or 'die-off' reaction. This occurs when the harmful microbes that are responsible for the gut dysbiosis (and therefore the symptoms) die. The dying microbes are broken down and release toxins (called endotoxins) that escape into the blood stream through the 'leaky gut'. These trigger the Ninja immune system and cause inflammation and therefore symptoms. This is another reason why I do not immediately introduce fermented foods in Phase I. The beneficial microbes may overwhelm and kill off the harmful microbes, so creating the die-off reaction. Although, for the most part, symptoms of die-off tend to be mild, this reaction can be quite serious. Symptoms can range from feeling fatigued to stomach cramps and diarrhoea, cold symptoms, a chest or urinary tract infection and rashes. In patients who already have a poor Ninja/immune response to illness, these reactions can be much more serious and potentially life-threatening. This is the reason why we follow the Diet to Detox in a step-by-step fashion. Slow and steady wins the day.

The second possible mechanism for non-linear progress to wellbeing is to do with toxins. In Phase I Diet to Detox we remove toxins from our food (and environment). When we stop presenting toxins to the body, this initially allows the gut to heal and allows the Ninja peas to begin to recover. The body may then decide that it is well enough to start to eliminate the toxins that are stored inside the body. Toxins can be stored in the liver, fatty tissues, organs, bones and the brain. If the body begins to mobilise these toxins, they will need to come into the blood stream, where their presence will be sensed by the specialised Ninja peas. When they are identified, this sparks an immune reaction which results in inflammation – the very thing that we are trying to deal with. If the levels of inflammation are still high, adding more inflammation will result in a worsening of the symptoms.

A third possible explanation I have for 'wavy recovery' is biofilms in the body. A biofilm is a combination of bacteria and yeasts (and other microbes) living in a mutually effective community. Biofilms are part of life, both in the body and in the environment. For those of you who are already familiar with kombucha, the SCOBY of the kombucha, which stands for Symbiotic Combination of Bacteria and Yeast, is a biofilm. The SCOBY is formed from multiple sheets of biofilm layers. The microbes live inside a matrix frame which is made up of polysaccharides or complex sugars. The biofilms are highly sturdy and resistant to damage. They often withstand antibiotics. In the human body the most well studied biofilms are to be found around the teeth, in the gut and on the skin, but they may also be in the lungs and the bladder. Each biofilm layer will have a particular characteristic depending on the environment that it lives in. The environment can be both physical and non-physical. That is to say, the biofilm development is dependent on the nutrients that are available to it. For example, if the environment contains mercury, your biofilm will adapt to be able to 'eat' or use mercury. These mercury-fixing microbes will then grow and multiply in the biofilm.

The non-physical environment will also determine the characteristic of microbes that are able to grow and multiply in the biofilm layer. When we think of the way the body works, we often think only of cells and enzyme processes. However, as mentioned in chapter 1, the body is electromagnetic. Our thoughts, feelings, stresses and worries also give off an electromagnetic frequency. These frequencies, just like food and toxins, will promote the growth and multiplication of certain classes of microbes. When we embark upon Phase I Diet to Detox, we begin to deprive the biofilms of physical toxins, which causes the microbes in that biofilm to die. The whole biofilm layer or layers that have this particular characteristic may then slough off. This process of biofilm layer removal may activate the Ninja peas, which as we know in turn produces inflammation, which in turn produces symptoms.

It can be easy to think that, just because the symptoms get worse, the programme isn't working or that your body is 'disagreeing' with a particular food. In fact, just the opposite may be occurring. The body may be 'waking up' and removing toxins, or a biofilm layer may be being discharged. I will talk more about what happens when biofilms are uncovered in the next chapter. I am also writing a biofilm module for my website *www.doctorese.com*.

HOW SHOULD I DEAL WITH WAVY REACTIONS?

One of the reasons that there are three phases in Diet to Detox is to avoid big peaks and troughs in the waves of recovery. At first, we just remove the toxins, then we introduce fermented food, then we reintroduce old friends. However, even just removing the toxins in Phase I Diet to Detox can produce a wavy reaction. It can be difficult to predict just who will undergo wavy recovery. As, mentioned above, in general, children tend to follow a more linear path. After the age of eighteen there seems to be more of a tendency to produce waves. I'd like to be able to say that the sicker you are or the more symptoms you have, the more waves you produce, but this isn't always the case. However, if I am faced with someone with a lot of symptoms or someone who is very reluctant to give up their favourite foods, I sometimes recommend a pre-Phase I Diet to Detox. This sometimes helps to dampen down the peak and troughs of the waves. According to my explanations above, what I think is happening here is that by slowing progress into Phase I, we slow down the rate that the body starts to eliminate body toxins. We may also slow down the breakdown of the biofilm layer. Both of these mechanisms result in lower levels of reactive inflammation and therefore fewer negative symptoms.

WHAT IS PRE-PHASE I DIET TO DETOX?

There is no hard and fast rule for a pre-Phase I. It just means that we introduce Phase I slowly. This could mean that we eliminate the culprit foods on just one day per week and the other six days we eat our normal diet. We then assess how we feel in the few days after the Diet to Detox day. If that one day makes you feel awful for the rest of the week, then you would stick to one day of pre-Phase I Diet to Detox until you no longer have a wavey reaction to it. If, on the other hand, you have no ill effects or mild effects that last just a few days, then the next week, you would do two days of Phase I Diet to Detox. Again, you would assess how well your system has coped with the two days of Phase I Diet to Detox. If it has responded with wavy symptoms you would stick to two days of Phase I until you no longer experience symptoms. If you have coped well with two days of Phase I, then the next week you increase the number of days on Phase I and so on, until you are doing Phase I Diet to Detox for seven days per week.

Another alternative way of doing a pre-Phase I is to choose one meal a day (at the same time each day) that is a Phase I Diet to Detox meal. This means you get to choose which meal that is. This might be breakfast. So, for example, if previously you were eating oats, yoghurts, nuts, seeds and berries, you would find a Phase I alternative from the recipes to replace these culprit foods. Lunch and dinner would be the same as you might normally have. If the thought of replacing your favourite breakfast is just too much, choose a different meal. You might also choose to start by replacing your culprit breakfast just at weekends or just for a few days per week. At the end of each day you would take a physical or mental note of how you feel having replaced the culprit meal. Once your body is no longer 'reacting' to the replacement meal, you are ready to move on.

Of course, you also need to feel emotionally ready to replace or modify the next meal. It came as a slight surprise to me just how emotive food can be. Taking away the comforting culprit meals, which of course is an oxymoron, can lead to some pretty dramatic reactions. Here I have a confession to make: I used to eat two croissants on the way to work. I would eat one at Brighton train station and then another at the coffee shop near my work off Oxford Street in London. When I first thought of following my own advice, I realised that I needed to get rid of croissants for breakfast. I would still drink a black coffee, but I stopped the croissants on my way to work. That short, three-minute walk from the coffee shop to my clinic became a cold and dark experience for six weeks. Then, almost overnight, the feelings of gloom were gone. I have never had a craving for those morning croissants again.

Before this time, I used to drink coffee with full cream milk. This combination is a delight! I loved the sharpness of the coffee and the creaminess of the milk. Of course, full cream milk is 'good' for you – full of good fats and protein. But as explained previously, the 'good' becomes 'bad' when the milk contains mycotoxins that are passed onto you from the cow that has been fed grains. The 'good' also becomes 'bad' when the grains fed to the cow have been sprayed with pesticides. I gave up the milk before the croissants, and this too was a miserable process. I tried alternatives such as soya, oat and almond milks (I didn't know about mould and pesticides in those days so didn't know that these alternatives were also culprit foods), but none of them tasted like full cream milk. Removing milk ruined my coffee drinking experience for months, but my energy levels and my lifelong eczema improved when I stopped milk and milk products.

I guess what I'm sharing here is just how attached we are to food. I find that now I use NMT, these strong attachment issues become less of a problem as I begin to deal with the root of this attachment.

The beauty of doing pre-Phase I Diet to Detox is that you have some control of what you give up first. If you combine this with dealing with MESS issues, then you are likely to have a much smoother ride.

During Phase I proper, I must stress that you should avoid even small amounts of the culprit foods. This is because, in order for the immune system to stop reacting to the toxins, they need a complete break from the foods that carry the toxins. The immune system is quite clever in that it only takes a small amount of the original culprit food before it reacts. And remember that the immune system will even react to portions of the culprit food that do not contain toxins. This means you may think that by eating toxin-free food you are OK, but the immune system will think that you are still eating toxin-containing food until you give it a chance to 'forget' that it is sensitive to that food. This is why a complete break is necessary.

Having said that, (there is always a 'but'), I have seen many people begin to respond well to eliminating toxins even during the pre-Phase I Diet to Detox, particularly if they are dealing with their MESS issues.

WHAT CAN I EAT?

This is the next question I get asked after sharing the culprit list with my patients. It's a great question. What's left to eat is a voyage of discovery that will lead to new realms of food and cooking. Bring it on!

FOODS YOU CAN EAT: THE GREEN 'EAT' LIST

Brassica vegetables – cabbage, cauliflower, sprouts
Root vegetables – Sweet potato, potato, yam, cassava, turnip, parsnip, swede, Jerusalem artichokes, turmeric, celeriac, kohlrabi, carrots, Konjac (noodles), radish, daikon radish
Green bananas and plantain
Mushrooms
Squash and pumpkin
Garlic and onions
Globe Artichokes
Fresh (not dried) herbs
Fresh (not dried) spices
Seaweed
Fresh or frozen green peas
Tomatoes
Aubergine
Bell peppers
Chilli peppers
Cucumbers
Lemons and limes

The first thing to remember is that many people live normal, fulfilled lives without many of the foods on the culprit list. The second thing to remember is that you only need to do it for six weeks. Remember the 'good tree–bad tree' analogy? The 'good' tree represents our 'good' gut microbes – those growing in the large intestine or colon – and the 'bad' tree represents the harmful microbes. To promote good colon health, we need to nourish our colon cells. Foods that nourish the colon cells are called prebiotic foods. Prebiotic foods are not the same as probiotic foods. Probiotic refers to microbes that are taken in from foods (or supplements). Prebiotic refers to nutrients that promote good colon health. Prebiotic foods are often the foods that we think of as foods with a good fibre content, like vegetables such as cabbage, cauliflower, broccoli and sprouts. During Phase I Diet to Detox, it is advisable to cook these prebiotic foods so as to make them easier to digest. If you have been sick for some time, you are likely to have gut dysbiosis (leaky gut) and raw vegetables will be difficult for the gut to deal with. Digesting and absorbing nutrients from raw food requires an intact and working intestinal system, with the intestinal lining cells closely packed together and a good profile of gut microbes. The leaky gut does not allow good digestion and allows 'alien' molecules to pass through into the body, alerting the Ninja peas which then create inflammation. The 'good' raw food becomes 'bad' because the gut cannot adequately metabolise them. In the leaky gut situation, the gut would prefer it if you pre-digested the food first. Cooking these vegetables until they are soft eases the digestion process.

WHAT ABOUT JUICING?

Many people have embarked upon juicing as a way of introducing a lot of good nutrients into their diet in one easy drink. Theoretically you could use non-culprit foods and put them in a juicer and, voila! All your goodness in one hit. But there are a couple of reasons why I am not a fan of juicing. The first is that we were not created to eat puréed food – babies do that and then they wean onto solid food. The second is that I often find that people either love their morning juice and it causes no after effects, or they've tried juicing and it 'hurts' their stomach, either causing pain or the onset of irritable bowel symptoms.

My understanding of this is as follows. Many 'good' vegetables such as beetroot, rhubarb, kale and spinach contain oxalates, as do other foods such as nuts, chocolate and bran. Oxalates are produced normally as a by-product of digestion and, under circumstances of health, the beneficial microbes will 'eat' oxalates, using them as fuel. This means that if you have a healthy gut microbiota, you can eat oxalate-containing foods without much negative after effect. However, if you have gut dysbiosis, some of the harmful microbes, including yeasts such as Candida, themselves produce oxalates. So, instead of mopping up any oxalates from the 'good' foods that you eat, the dysbiotic microbes produce more, giving you a level of oxalates that creates problems in your body. For example, oxalates can combine with calcium to form calcium oxalate, which can be deposited in joints and cause gout-like pain and swelling. Calcium oxalate can also be deposited in muscles and tendons, causing stiffness and pain similar to the symptoms of fibromyalgia, or in the arteries, contributing to a hardening of the arteries and possibly leading to cardiovascular disease (which in turn causes strokes and heart attacks). As if that wasn't enough, calcium oxalate is also the main component of kidney stones.

So, you can understand that juicing, even with 'good' vegetables, can have some 'bad' effects. As many of my patients have gut dysbiosis, I tend to put juicing to one side until they have completed the programme and have no symptoms and are passing three soft stools per day. You could theoretically boil your non-culprit, low oxalate vegetables and put these in your juicer. This, of course, would be called soup! Joking aside, boiling oxalate-containing vegetables is a good way to eat them as the boiling process causes the oxalates to come out of the vegetables and into the water, which is then thrown away.

A WORD ABOUT CARBS

Sweet potatoes and potatoes are root vegetables and good prebiotic colon food. However, be careful. Just because they are on the 'good' list, doesn't mean that you should eat lots of them. If you are starting on this journey and you are overweight, eating lots of these root vegetables will lead to weight gain, so avoid eating too many root vegetables if you are overweight. If you are slim or underweight you may need to eat more of these types of vegetables, as well as protein, to maintain your weight. On my website *www.doctorese.com* I have a module entitled 'Sugars and Fasting', where I explain a practical way to find out how much 'white', blood sugar-raising/weight-enhancing carbohydrates you should eat.

WHAT ABOUT FATS?

Are fats 'good' or 'bad'? I'm sure by now you'll know that the answer isn't a simple one. Fats can be both 'good' and 'bad'. There is a trend at present to shun animal fats. This is a big rabbit hole to go down, so I will deal with just the wellbeing aspects and not the geopolitical aspects of this debate.

In their natural state, cows, sheep and goats like to eat grass. When they eat grass, they produce 'good' fat. When they are fed grains, however, they put on excess weight, which might be appealing to us as the consumer, but the fat they produce is 'bad' fat. Not only that, but the grain the animal is fed is likely to carry toxins from pesticides and moulds. So, not only is the fat a 'bad' type of fat, but it also will pass toxins down to us in the food chain. Most meat in the shops will not detail what the animal has been fed unless it has been fed a grass diet. Saturated fat (lard) from a grass-fed animal has health-giving properties and will help to lower inflammation. Fat-soluble vitamins (A, D, E, K) are essential for health, especially the gut, bones and brain. Most of us know that eating a diet rich in vegetables will provide us with plenty of good nutrients, including vitamins. However, what many do not know is that the vitamins – particularly the fat-soluble variety – will not be adequately absorbed into our body unless they are eaten with fat. Carrots are said to be a good source of vitamin A (the fat-soluble vitamin that helps you to see in the dark), but did you know that unless the carrot is grated into small strips and covered in oil, the fat-soluble vitamin A will not be available for the body to use? A better source of vitamin A is from oils such as sustainably sourced, raw, red palm oil and animal meats.

VITAMIN A
Eggs
Liver
Cod Liver
Sustainably sourced, raw red palm oil

Bones in particular need a good source of Vitamin D and Vitamin K2 – even more than they need calcium. Vitamin D, K2 and A are friends and work in tandem. Vitamin D and A cause absorption of calcium from the gut and, in order to get calcium into the bones, we need vitamin K2. A rich source of vitamin K2 is foie gras (force-fed goose liver), but don't shoot the messenger! I hear that there are now ethical sources of foie gras. Another rich source of vitamin K2 is a Japanese dish called Natto, which is made from fermented soyabeans. Fermented soyabeans are 'good'; non-fermented soyabeans are not. Natto is not to everyone's taste and consistency but with some imagination it can be incorporated into the diet. Emu oil is also another good source of vitamin K2, as are Swiss cheeses made from milk from grass-fed cows, but these should be avoided in Phase I Diet to Detox because of the potential milk-toxin cross-reactivity I mentioned previously. Remember, the Ninja peas will pick up on the milk part of the food and think that it is associated with the toxin. Avoiding the milk in Phase I allows the Ninja immune system to 'forget' that milk is a problem.

So, combining vegetables with good oils from grass-fed meat is a good way to get the best out of the nutrients in the vegetables. In this way, in Phase I Diet to Detox, your meals are likely to be mainly vegetables with a garnish of meat and plenty of other 'good' fats.

POLYUNSATURATED LIQUID OILS

Omega-3 oils from fish are particularly helpful at reducing inflammation. Before the days of ibuprofen (Advil in the US), cod liver oil was a treatment for painful joints. Lard (from a grass-fed cow) and virgin coconut oil can be used for cooking – including frying – as they are stable at high temperatures. Oils that are liquid at room temperature are not stable at high temperatures and therefore should not be used for high temperature cooking. The liquid oils, such as vegetable oil, olive oil, avocado oil etc, are marketed as being 'healthy' because of their omega-3, polyunsaturated fat content. However, the chemical structure of the bonds in polyunsaturated fats are inherently weak. This means that, not only are they not stable at high temperatures, but they are also unstable when exposed to sunlight. Being 'unstable' means that their bond structure easily breaks down. In real life, this means that they go 'off' or rancid if exposed to extremes of temperature. This might happen whilst the oil is stored in the warehouse or in transit or on the supermarket shelf. The going 'off' process or the break-up of the bonds during cooking produces inflammation-inducing free radicals. For this reason liquid oils should be kept in dark containers, preferably cans, and they should be stored in a cool place. When you visit countries that typically use olive oil, such as Greece and Italy, you find that the oil is stored in a cool place in the cellar. When I lived in the South of France, our local shop produced its own olive oil. This olive oil was cloudy and, when it was particularly cool, you could see blobs of lard floating in it. I suspect that these blobs of saturated fat keep the unsaturated fat stable, and this may be the reason why these traditional societies have no qualms about cooking with their olive oil.

POLY AND MONO-UNSATURATED FATS
Fish oil
Flax seed and oil
Avocado and oil
Olives and oil

So which olive oil should you buy? Search around and ask friends, who come from olive oil growing countries, where they get their olive oil. For the reasons mentioned above, please do throw away your oils labelled as 'vegetable oils'. There is nothing good to found in these oils. They are generally made using base products such as soya beans, rapeseed (canola), cottonseed, sunflower and corn. All of these fit nicely into the 'culprit food' list. They are likely to produce free radicals when cooked and are likely to contain toxins from the growing or storage phases. I have found that when patients replace just this one thing, many symptoms go away.

A QUICK WORD ABOUT CHOLESTEROL

Cholesterol is required to transport fats and other nutrients around the body, so it is actually a good thing. It also forms part of the wrapping around nerve sheaths. When you have a blood test and the 'bad' (LDL) cholesterol is raised, most doctors will tell you that this is because you are eating too much fat. This is not true. There is plenty of research that proves this, but mainstream medicine is just taking a very long time to catch up. Cholesterol is an antioxidant that responds to inflammation, so when the 'bad' cholesterol is raised it means that you have inflammation. The response, therefore, should be to deal with the inflammation rather than to deal with the cholesterol. Dealing with the cholesterol is like trying to stop the firefighters from getting to the fire. Dealing with the inflammation will mean that you won't need to take cholesterol-lowering drugs for the rest of your life.

Eggs and liver are a rich source of cholesterol. Eggs should be from chickens that have roamed outside and can peck and eat worms. Remember, chickens are not vegetarians – they eat meat (worms). How a chicken is reared and housed affects the quality and taste of the egg (5) (6). A happy chicken that lives a normal life produces 'happy' eggs. An unhappy, stressed chicken, on the other hand, will produced 'stressed' eggs that contain 'stress' molecules that might just get passed to us when we eat them.

SIGNS OF PROGRESS IN PHASE I DIET TO DETOX

The body uses several mechanisms to get rid of toxic waste. These are detailed below:

DETOXIFICATION MECHANISMS
Gut/liver
Kidneys
Lungs
Sweating

Ideally, all of these detoxification pathways should be working well, but the most important of these mechanisms, for our purposes, is the gut–liver pathway. This is because we can clearly see when our bowel habit is changing. Remember, the optimum number of bowel openings should be two to three per day of soft, reasonably large stools. If your stools are too loose, this could represent a need for a more diverse population of gut microbes. A happy gut is also one with little gas and certainly no pain. It is normal to open the bowels soon after waking and after each meal.

Drinking 'good' water will assist urine detoxification via the kidneys. We talked about some of the toxins in tap water in chapter 4, so use a good filtration system that also gives energy to the water. Space doesn't allow me to expand upon this topic, but you can find out more about water on my website *www.doctorese.com.*

The lungs and our breath are of course vital for the good exchange of oxygen and carbon dioxide. But we also use our lungs in a similar way to the liver. The lungs detoxify our bodies from toxins such as moulds and plastics, just like the liver does (7) (8). So what happens if we don't breathe properly? During my consultations, I teach people how to breathe via their abdomen and not using their shoulders and upper chest. I find that the 'hunched shoulder' way of holding oneself is common and brings with it not only poor breathing but a holding-on of emotions. The simple task of learning to breathe from the abdomen often releases emotion. Remember that we are electromagnetic beings. Emotions are stored as electromagnetic frequency signatures in our body water. I have only experience of my own practice to suggest that when we learn to breathe properly, we allow the release of emotions which are tied to the body's ability to hold on to toxins. When we release the emotions, we can release the toxins, which then helps us to heal.

Sweating comes when we exercise or sit somewhere hot, like a sauna. The heat that is produced allows toxins that are sitting in our tissues to be released, so we must always be sure to drink good water and shower after exercise to complete the elimination process. The smell of our sweat may change as we detoxify. Allowing the body to sweat each day is a good practice. However, if you are very sick, exercising may initially make you feel worse as it creates inflammation. I advise people to listen to their body when deciding how much exercise to do. If, after five minutes of a light stroll, you have a mild sweat, then this is sufficient. If it takes an hour of vigorous sprints to produce a mild sweat then this is sufficient for you. Of, course if you have a joint problem, doing an hour of vigorous physical activity may harm the already injured joint. You may then need to choose other methods, such as a hot sauna or an infra-red sauna to allow you to sweat. Be careful, however, as too much sweating may result in too much detoxification. If your bowels and lungs are not working as well as they should, you may not eliminate all of the toxins you have released from the tissues. If the gut and lungs are not working well, the released toxins will trigger the Ninja immune system to create inflammation and you will then feel unwell. The incomplete elimination process then means that the toxins go back to their original hiding place, which means that you have to go through the elimination process all over again once all of the detoxification pathways are working.

SUGGESTED COMBINATIONS FOR MEALS IN PHASE I DIET TO DETOX

With a long list of 'culprit foods' off the menu, mealtimes in Phase I might seem tricky. Here are some suggested food combinations for meals:

BREAKFAST

Fish
Naturally fed sausages, bacon or other meat leftovers from dinner
Eggs
Vegetables, cooked until soft
Avocado
Mushrooms of all edible varieties. Try marinading them in garlic oil then frying in coconut oil.

DRINKS

Filtered water
Hot coconut milk and blackstrap molasses (black treacle)

LUNCHES AND DINNERS

When planning lunches and dinners, be aware of your weight and whether you need to lose or maintain it. Root vegetables and other fibre-rich foods have wonderful prebiotic properties, and if you are slim and need to maintain weight, then go ahead and eat these foods at any meal. However, they will raise glucose and insulin levels, which can lead to weight gain, so if you need to lose weight they should be eaten either in the morning or in the middle of the day. This gives time for your mitochondria to recover. Eating them late at night will not give time for the mitochondria to be refreshed.

If you are eating these foods just once per day in the morning or at midday but still find that you are overweight, then you need to reduce the amount that you eat at these meals. You can find more information on this in the 'Sugars and Fasting' module on my website *www.doctorese.com*. The prebiotic vegetables that can lead to weight gain in some people include: yams, cassava, green and yellow plantain, potatoes, sweet potato, squash, pumpkin, celeriac, swedes and turnips.

STARTERS

Try a simple soup starter of slow-cooked vegetables with garlic and fresh herbs. Try adding some good oils to the soup, such as coconut oil, olive oil or red palm oil (just a little, as too much can be overwhelming unless you are making a tomato soup).

If you are feeling a little under the weather you could try a stronger soup such as garlic or mushroom soup or try the recipe for Dr Ese's Detox soup in the recipe section.

Seaweed and garlic is another great starter to get the gastric juices flowing and provides minerals and iodine as well as the anti-inflammatory garlic.

Mushrooms again are another good way to introduce anti-inflammatory molecules. Remember, if you give them a little soak in the sun on the windowsill for a few hours, they will make their own vitamin D.

MAIN COURSES

During Diet to Detox Phase I your main meal will consist mostly of meat and vegetables. Try cooking the vegetables until soft and then tossing in some gently warmed garlic oil or just plain olive oil with fresh herbs and salt.

You could also try slow cooked vegetables of your choice or a roasted vegetable medley. Squash cut in half and cooked slowly with added garlic oil and fresh herbs is a simple yet delicious vegetable option.

Try slow cooking your meat too, including chicken, lamb, pork, beef, duck and game. If you have no problem with nightshade vegetables, you could make a mixed tomato and aubergine relish with fresh herbs and salt.

Fish and coconut are an easy combination. You can take fish from the freezer and add coconut milk or coconut cream and throw in some fresh herbs or fresh turmeric to give it an exotic twist. If you can get it, some fresh fenugreek leaves are another nice addition. Be careful to use coconut milk with as few additives as possible – cans tend to have fewer than cartons. Japanese Konjac noodles make a great addition to this dish. They are a root vegetable with very little calorific value so are great if you are trying not to gain weight.

DESSERTS

I'm afraid that desserts are limited in Phase I Diet to Detox. You could, however, try some blackstrap molasses. Blackstrap molasses, or black treacle, is a wonder sugar that doesn't behave like a sugar at all. Molasses not only provides a range of minerals and vitamins, but it also binds toxins, so the more toxins you have in your system, the more molasses you need. I often recommend taking molasses like a supplement. I've noticed that when the body is carrying a lot of toxins, some people will need over ten dessert spoons per day of blackstrap molasses. And there is no weight gain! Understanding how much blackstrap molasses you need is a clever but simple process. If you experience constipation, you need more blackstrap molasses. Keep increasing the amount of molasses you take until the constipation or infrequent passing of hard stools stops and you are having three soft stools per day. Once you begin to get rid of the toxins, the amount of blackstrap molasses you need will go down and you may find that you need only one dessert spoon or less per day.

You can eat blackstrap molasses neat from a spoon, heated with coconut milk, which makes a type of fudge or, if you have an ice cream maker, you can make a delicious ice cream with coconut milk or coconut cream.

CHAPTER 7

PHASE II DIET TO DETOX: HEALING WITH FERMENTATION

If the aim of Phase I Diet to Detox is to eliminate toxins, then the aim of Phase II is to strengthen the gut. We can do this through fermented foods. First, let's briefly recap upon why we need fermented foods in our lives. Fermented foods are colon food – in other words, the probiotics in fermented foods are like friends to our colon cells, helping to strengthen both the cells and the gap junctions. This means that they help to heal the 'leaky gut'. This process will have already started when you removed the toxins from the diet and environment in Phase I, but by introducing fermented foods you will allow this to improve further.

Fermented food, of course, does so much more than help repair the 'leaky gut'. Here are some other areas that are improved by fermentation:

'Colon food'	helps repair the 'leaky gut'
Digestion	provides enzymes that help to breakdown carbs, proteins and fats
Nutrients	helps provide vitamins such as folate, B1, 2, 3, 6, 12, K2
Antimicrobial	helps to fight infection from viruses, bacteria and yeasts
Detoxification	helps to remove toxins
Anti-cancer	helps to prevent cancers from forming
Immune function	helps to re-establish a functional immune system

If you are not eating a range of fermented foods, you are missing out on this whole list of amazing benefits. Who wouldn't want to help their body digest food, gain more nutrients from foods instead of supplements, fight infection, get rid of harmful toxins, prevent cancer and make sure that the immune system is working as it should?

Eating fermented food is not just about taking in a natural

probiotic and adding to your gut microbes. In the fermentation module on my website *www.doctorese.com*, I describe the 'fermentation equation'. This describes what happens when a culture of microbes in the form of a ferment is given fuel in the form of sugar or protein. The culture of beneficial, probiotic microbes utilises the sugar or protein as fuel and the microbes multiply. But this isn't all. They also produce wonderful bioactive substances, including vitamins and digestive enzymes.

Some ferments, like shiokoji, a rice ferment from Japan, also produce peptides, which are small strings of protein that behave like hormones in the body. Peptides are particularly relevant at the moment, as I recently discovered. I buy shiokoji by the boxful from my friend Yasuko's shop, Kantenya in Brighton, UK. One day, not long ago, I asked for my usual supply and Yasuko told me that she would need to ration how much she gave me because the suppliers were sending less and less from Japan. When I asked why, she told me it was because scientists had discovered that microbes associated with fermented cabbage may help to prevent infection from COVID 19. Indeed, a search through the academic literature confirms this (9, 10).

Another rice ferment product called sake lees is also rich in bioactive peptides. Sake lees is made from the left-over fermented rice, yeasts and other by-products after making Japanese sake beer. Sake lees contains at least nine peptides that can prevent infection through the nasal passages and lungs.

At the outset of the coronavirus alert in 2020, whilst the West saw a run on toilet paper, Japan saw a run on Natto, the fermented soyabean product. It also appears that the areas of Japan that consume Natto had lower death rates from COVID-19. Indeed, studies have shown that low vitamin K2 may play a role in the causation of blood clots that contribute to COVID-19 deaths (11) and, as we know, Natto is rich in vitamin K2.

WHICH FOODS ARE FERMENTED?

VEGETABLES
PROTEINS
DESSERTS
DRINKS

I've mentioned previously that when I mention the words 'fermented foods', most people have a limited idea of what I mean. But 'fermented foods' cover almost every main food category, including vegetables, proteins, desserts and drinks.

Understanding what causes fermentation in our food can be a little daunting, but it is important to be aware of how the fermentation process comes about and what wonderful products are created by the microbes.

WINE

Most fresh foods will undergo some sort of fermentation given the right conditions. Think about grapes that make wine. In the old days, wine producers did not use a specific yeast, such as *Saccharomyces Cerevisiae,* to bring about the fermentation process – they would rely on the yeasts that naturally lived on the fruit to ferment the grape. There is a move to return to these old ways of fermentation. However, the downside of this organic process is that you get a highly variable end product – some wines will be great and others not so great.

SAUERKRAUT AND KIMCHI

Traditional sauerkraut is made by adding salt to cabbage and allowing the natural microbes on the surface of the cabbage to ferment it. The salt helps the process because it naturally kills off unwanted microbes. The Koreans use this method to make kimchi. This version of naturally fermented cabbage uses salt but also adds other ingredients such as pepper and chillies to give a spicy, piquant flavour to the cabbage. The spices also result in the production of additional bioactive substances.

SHIOKOJI

In Japan, rather than using the natural microbes on the cabbage to make sauerkraut, they add shiokoji. *Shio* means salt and *Koji* means culture. In this case, the culture or ferment is made from rice. If you haven't noticed already, this book has a strong Japanese influence. The Japanese have a long history of food research and understand its importance for health. They also happen to be amongst the longest-lived people of the developed nations and Japan has the highest number of Michelin-starred restaurants, second only to France. My Japanese friend Yasuko told me that the focus of food research in Japan was often to find the most health-giving foods to serve to the Emperor. Once the Emperor was known to eat a certain food, then the rest of the population would follow suit. shiokoji is a well-researched ferment and is used a lot in Japanese cooking. Yasuko taught me all about this wonderful ferment and I feel honoured to pass on her knowledge to you through this book.

KEFIR
Kefir is a fermented milk drink made with a combination of different yeasts and bacteria to bring about fermentation. It can be made with coconut milk as well as dairy milk and was originally stored in goatskin bags.

KOMBUCHA
Kombucha is a lightly sparkling fermented green or black tea that uses a wide range of different yeasts and bacteria to achieve fermentation.

FERMENT BLEND
I have also developed my own multipurpose ferment, called *Ferment Blend,* that can be used to ferment a wide variety of foods including chocolate, yoghurts and breads.

SHIOKOJI
KEFIR
KOMBUCHA
FERMENT BLEND

HOW TO INTRODUCE FERMENTED FOOD
To avoid the 'wavy' reaction to fermented food we talked about in chapter 6, you should introduce new fermented foods slowly. My usual recommendation is to introduce one new food per week. One week can be 5-7 days, depending on any reactions you may have. Remember that reactions can vary from a mild sense of fatigue through to abdominal pain, bloating and diarrhoea or even chest infection and flu-like symptoms. The symptoms may be brief, lasting just a few hours, or may continue for a number of weeks. It is impossible to predict who will get these reactions, which is why I recommend proceeding with care during Phase II of Diet to Detox.

I also normally recommend a particular order in which to

introduce the foods to cause as little upset to the system as possible. Luckily, there is a stage *before* fermented food called pre-fermentation.

PRE-FERMENTED MEATS

I recommend that you start by 'pre-fermenting' meat, fish or chicken by marinating it in a fermented product before cooking it. My preferred ferment for this process is – in case you hadn't guessed – shiokoji. Ferment the meat for 8-12 hours or overnight and then cook it as you normally would. I call this *pre-fermentation* because the shiokoji starts to digest the meat so that your intestines have less work to do. This also means that there are fewer waste products for your intestines and liver to deal with. And of course, the fermentation means that many wonderful bioactive substances are produced. Most of the probiotic microbes are killed during cooking, but not all, as some lactic acid bacteria are able to survive high-temperature cooking. This means that you'll get some probiotic microbes but not too many – ideal when you are first introducing fermented foods. You will also get additional bioactive substances such as vitamins and the powerful, hormone-like peptides. If there is no 'wavy' reaction to pre-fermented cooked meat, you can than progress on to pre-fermented cooked vegetables.

PRE-FERMENTED VEGETABLES

For the vegetable phase, you might choose almost any green or colourful vegetable or mushrooms. Again, I tend to use shiokoji to pre-ferment vegetables before cooking them. If you can't easily get hold of shiokoji, try using water kefir. Sweet potatoes, squash and pumpkin don't do so well using shiokoji as they tend to become discoloured and unappealing, but other vegetables such as cabbage, bell peppers, aubergines, onions, spring onions, leeks, cauliflower and courgettes do well being pre-fermented in shiokoji for 4-12 hours before cooking. Cook them until they are soft, as you did in Phase I. Mushrooms, pre-fermented in shiokoji and olive oil for 4-8 hours then pan fried in coconut oil until soft, are divine. I discovered this recipe myself and offered some to Yasuko to get her verdict. She loved them! I didn't eat mushrooms much before I discovered this way of preparing them, but it is so simple and delicious that now I eat them all the time.

At this point, mid-way through Phase II Diet to Detox, it can be tempting to throw a whole load of vegetables in a pot at the same time and jump into fermentation with all your might, but resist this temptation. It is best to maintain the slow and steady pace and choose just one vegetable per week, as you may find that you are OK with certain vegetables but not others. This is where you really need to be patient with the process. Going too quickly at this stage can make you ill for a number of weeks, which can be so demoralising that you give up. Better to go slowly and make your way back to a wonderful state of wellness than be over-eager and derail your progress.

Interestingly, I find that broccoli is one of the most troublesome vegetables for those who have had 'leaky gut'. It is best to leave this vegetable to towards the end of Phase II. Many people are also concerned if they have had previous reactions to nightshade vegetables (tomatoes, aubergine, bell peppers and potatoes). In my experience, pre-fermentation before cooking can get rid of reactions to these foods in some people. If nightshades have been a problem for you, perhaps leave them to end of Phase II or even Phase III, as this will give your gut even more time to restore itself before tackling them.

DESSERTS

Once you have introduced a few new pre-fermented vegetables, you may choose to continue to add more pre-fermented vegetables. Or, if you can't wait to reintroduce something sweet, you may opt for desserts! The easiest dessert to make is fermented coconut milk with molasses (black treacle). You can use either coconut milk kefir or my Ferment Blend to ferment the coconut milk. You can often buy coconut milk yoghurts from the shops, but be careful with these. They are often *cultured* and not fermented. What's the difference? *Cultured* often means that the microbes are added to the milk just before they put the lid on, giving no time for fermentation to happen and so no time for the microbes to digest the milk or produce wonderful bioactive substances. Also, if you buy the milk from the shop and the sugar that is used in the ferment is a refined sugar, you will also be eating refined sugar (even though some will be used in the fermentation equation). If shop-bought yoghurt is all you have and you cannot make your own, what you can do is open the lid to allow some oxygen into the yoghurt. Rest the lid back on top of the yoghurt and then leave the yoghurt out on the countertop for 8-12 hours, depending on the temperature in your kitchen, before consuming. You will know that fermentation is taking place because you will start to see bubbles forming in it and the taste will become tart rather than sweet.

RAW FERMENTED VEGETABLES

Once you've tried pre-fermented meats and vegetables and a simple yoghurt, you can then go on to even more ferments, for example raw fermented vegetables. For this, you can use either shiokoji or water kefir. Soft cabbage, such as the cabbage used to make kimchi (napa cabbage), or pointy cabbage are good beginner cabbages. These fermented cabbage dishes taste nothing like sauerkraut. They are much milder and not at all acidic if you eat them within 24 hours. However, they will keep for weeks in a jar in the fridge and will then become more and more sour as time goes on.

By this stage you should be eating a range of pre-fermented vegetables, so there should be no need to choose just one raw ferment per week. You can now combine different vegetables and create a raw fermented vegetable medley.

RAW FERMENTED FISH

Once you have introduced some raw fermented vegetables, you could try raw fermented fish. Most people look aghast when I mention fermented fish. They simply can't imagine such a food and think that it must smell awful. In fact, this could not be further from the truth. Fish such as salmon or trout can be combined with a dash of shiokoji and some coconut milk to make a scrumptious fish mousse. These fish ferments are delicious to have as a starter or a side dish and are so simple to make. They will last for weeks, fermenting away in the fridge. Although, really, they won't last that long.

FERMENTED DRINKS

We have already introduced kefir to the fermentation process. Kefir water or coconut kefir is refreshing when combined with fresh ginger, fresh mint or lemons and limes. Try these first before moving on to kombucha, as you'll remember that it can create a powerful 'die off' reaction as it did in my son Luke. For some people, just a few teaspoons of kombucha can cause a 'wavy' reaction. Start by taking just one teaspoon of kombucha then reassess how you feel the next day. If all is well, double the amount and continue to double the amount each day until you can manage a whole glass.

KOMBUCHA SALADS

Once you can manage a glass of kombucha, you are ready to make kombucha salads. These are so simple. Take the chopped

> ROUTE MAP THROUGH PHASE II DIET TO DETOX
> *Pre-fermented then cooked meat*
> *Pre-fermented then cooked vegetables*
> *A simple dessert*
> *Raw fermented vegetables using shiokoji or water kefir*
> *Fermented fish*
> *Fermented drinks*
> *Kombucha fermented vegetables*

vegetable, add a splash of kombucha, a glug of olive oil, salt and pepper and that's it! The first time I made a kombucha vegetable ferment, I used tomatoes and I was amazed that they were transformed into a gourmet delight. In fact, fermentation with kombucha truly transforms almost all vegetables. Even slightly tart vegetables become sweet within about four hours, and I've found that children who previously turned their noses up at vegetables will gobble these up. Remember not to skip the oil, as this not only lends a softer feel to the vegetables but also allows you to absorb more wonderful bioactive substances. The salt and pepper are a must also, as they bring out the flavour in the vegetables.

If the pathway for Phase II Diet to Detox above seems a little strict, it's because I felt that it was important to give a clear pathway for those who are truly sick and do not have access to help. When I consult with patients one-to-one, I often see them on a weekly basis so I can direct them as to which food to introduce the following week. By making Phase II so prescriptive, I hope that it gives you a clear route through to Phase III without needing my individual help.

WHAT DO I DO IF I HAVE A 'WAVY' REACTION WHEN I INTRODUCE A FERMENTED FOOD?

You may have a true allergy to a food. If you are an adult, you are likely to already be aware of which foods you are allergic to, so if you have a true allergy to a particular food, please do continue to avoid it. As explained in the previous chapter, the 'wavy' reaction can be due to a number of possible reactions that your body may have. These include:

- A 'die off' reaction
- Toxin release
- Biofilm breakdown

If you start to feel unwell after eating a certain food and your reaction involves the following symptoms – shortness of breath, itching lips, mouth or throat, a rash or redness – it is likely to represent a true allergic reaction, so seek emergency medical help. You may need antihistamine and corticosteroid medication to settle the reaction. The reactions above are rare, however, and usually happen with an already known food allergen.

The 'wavy' type of reaction that I first explained in the previous chapter may vary from immediate symptoms such as fatigue, abdominal cramps and diarrhoea or may come on after a few hours and make you feel more systemically unwell with a chest infection, cold or flu-like symptoms, a rash or even urinary

One reason some people feel unwell after the introduction of fermented foods is that microbes from the probiotic food may pass through a 'leaky gut' into the body. In people that are especially immunocompromised, the gut may be slow to heal and introducing fermented foods may allow 'good' microbes into the blood stream. Probiotic microbes are not supposed to enter the blood stream; they are supposed to stay in the gut. Once inside the body, they can cause serious illness. One example of a 'good' probiotic turned 'bad' is Saccharomyces Cerevisiae and its relative Saccharomyces Boulardii. Most of us have heard of Candida (Albicans). We know this is a 'bad' microbe. You may know that it causes a condition called thrush either in the mouth or in the genital area. In these situations, the Candida is growing on the mucosal surface and is not inside the body. Invasive Candida Albicans, on the other hand, is a severe condition whereby the yeast gains access to the body and even the brain to cause serious disease (12). In the immunocompromised individual, if yeasts like Saccharomyces Cerevisiae and Saccharomyces Boulardii enter the blood stream, they can cause severe disease that is indistinguishable from a severe systemic candida infection (13) (14). An invasive yeast infection such as these requires intravenous anti-fungal medication for treatment. It is for this reason that I recommend a slow and steady pace for Phase II of Diet to Detox. If you find that you are having one 'wavy' reaction after the other and this is coupled by debilitating symptoms such as severe fatigue and there are no road blocks, the possibility of moderate or severe immunocompromise should be borne in mind.

symptoms that appear to be a urinary tract infection. As mentioned above, these 'wavy' reactions may be due to a 'die off', toxin release or possibly biofilm breakdown. In Chapter 5, I also mentioned another important factor that can cause a reaction after eating fermented food in particular. It is when 'good' microbes leak through the gut.

The ideal situation during Phase II is that you introduce fermented foods without any reactions and no return of symptoms together with an ongoing improved sense of wellbeing. But if you do suffer from a 'wavy' reaction, the first thing to do is to stop eating that food and take note of the duration and severity of the reaction.

In terms of duration, the reaction may last for:

- just a few hours – mild
- a few days – moderate
- a few weeks – severe

In terms of severity, the reaction may be:

- mild e.g. you can still go about your daily activities
- moderate e.g. you have to reduce your daily activities
- severe e.g. you have to stop your usual routine and take to your bed or seek medical help

Usually, if a reaction is mild in duration, it is also mild in severity. Here are some suggestions for what to do if you have mild/mild, moderate/moderate or severe/severe reactions.

MILD/MILD REACTIONS.
If both duration and severity are mild, wait until the symptoms have calmed down and re-try the food for a further week. If the symptoms no longer return, then you are free to continue eating this food. If the symptoms return, remove this food from your 'can eat list' and retry it at a later date, in say 2+ weeks' time.

MODERATE/MODERATE REACTIONS.
Remove this food from your 'can eat list' and retry after 6+ weeks. If, when you retry it, you again have a reaction, either wait another three months or generally avoid it.

SEVERE/SEVERE REACTION.
Remove this food from the 'can eat list' and re-try a very tiny

portion, such as half a teaspoon, in three months' time. If, when you re-try it, you again have a reaction, either wait another three months or generally avoid it.

Not all reactions will follow the patterns I've just described. For example, you may experience severe stomach cramps, bloating and diarrhoea for just a few hours. You may need to stop what you are doing and rest for those few hours but after that you are able to resume your normal activities. In this situation I feel that it is safest to act on the most severe rating and remove the food for at least three months before trying it again in a very small dose.

By the end of Phase II Diet to Detox, you should be enjoying a full and varied menu of delicious, nutrient-dense foods. If you have taken the slow and steady route, you should also now be ready to start reintroducing old friends back into your life.

SUGGESTED FOOD COMBINATIONS FOR MEALS IN PHASE II DIET TO DETOX

Try to include some fermented food in each meal but remember, start slowly.

BREAKFASTS

Fermented coconut milk yoghurt.
Fish, either pre-fermented or raw fermented.
Naturally fed pre-fermented sausages, bacon or other meat leftovers from dinner.
Eggs. Try eggs fermented overnight with shiokoji.
Avocado.
Full range of vegetables, either pre-fermented or raw fermented.
Pre-fermented mushrooms of all edible varieties.
Drinks
Good water
Molasses and coconut milk
Kombucha and kefir

LUNCHES AND DINNERS

Remember that if you are trying to lose weight you will need to avoid root vegetables such as yams, cassava, green and yellow plantain, potatoes, sweet potato, squash, pumpkin, celeriac, swedes and turnips, or restrict them to the morning or middle of the day.

STARTERS

Pre-fermented vegetable soup with added good oils, or pre-fermented garlic soup or Dr Ese's Detox soup for days when you need a boost.

Pre-fermented seaweed and garlic starter.

Pre-fermented mushrooms soaked in some garlic oil, then fried very gently in coconut oil.

MAIN COURSES

Pre-fermented vegetables tossed in some gently warmed garlic oil.

Pre-fermented and cooked vegetables of your choice or a roasted vegetable medley.

Pre-fermented and cooked meats including chicken, lamb, pork, beef and duck. How about combining pre-fermented ribs with a fermented tomato relish, or a fermented marmalade with duck. The fermented marmalade also goes well with fermented cabbage.

A pre-fermented fish and coconut stew as per Phase I, combined with Konjac or Kanten noodles.

DESSERTS

Fermented coconut yoghurt with lemon or lime.

Kombucha or kefir sorbet with lemon or lime and blackstrap molasses.

Sake lees and coconut milk ice-cream. Adding sake lees makes such an amazingly expensive-tasting ice cream that you'll never want to eat shop-bought ice cream again.

CHAPTER 8

PHASE III DIET TO DETOX: REINTRODUCING AND MAINTENANCE

Phase III of Diet to Detox is the grand finale. At this point in the programme your body should feel great. You have removed toxins from your food and environment and the addition of fermented food has further strengthened the gut and immune system. Now you get to reintroduce old friends.

Like in Phase II, I have a particular set of suggestions for how you should reintroduce those old culprit foods. Hopefully by now the body no longer recognises the food itself as toxic and has forgotten that it was previously associated with harmful molecules.

A WORD OF CAUTION

There is a 'but' here. When you reintroduce old friends, if you reintroduce the exact same foods as you did previously and there are toxins in those foods, you will be starting the whole process all over again. Here's an example of how this can happen. After Phase II we are feeling on top form and fancy a few oats for breakfast, like in the old days. We have a bowl of oats and coconut yoghurt and still feel good. The next week perhaps we decide to add some fresh fruit and then nuts into the mix and we still feel great. We think we've cracked it – we've returned to wellbeing. Then, just slowly, we get that odd twinge in the tummy whilst eating certain foods or we begin to get a little constipated, or the joints feel a little achy. And before we know it, more and more symptoms have come back. What has happened? Of course, we are back to square one. And why wouldn't we be? We are again eating culprit foods. We have again taken on board enough toxins to injure our gut, create dysbiosis, trigger the Ninja peas and develop inflammation.

This scenario happens all too often. So what can we do to prevent this slide back to square one? My first piece of advice is to choose your friends wisely. You may be desperate to reintroduce oats but think about finding a version that is free from mycotoxins and pesticides. This, of course, may not be possible. If this is the case, then by all means see that friend once in a while but perhaps not all the time. When you reintroduce oats, you may be fine the first time, the second time and even for many weeks, but eventually the toxins will build up again. So try not to eat the same culprit food every day. Switch things around a little bit and include some variety in what you eat. You might think of eating oats just at the weekends, rather than every day. In this way, you are less likely to see a return of old symptoms.

Always have a large side of fermented vegetables of your liking. Try to vary this so that your body gets a look at different types of microbes. You could combine fermented cabbage with nuts or currants and for added flavour throw in some coriander or North African sumac. The herbs give an added depth to the vegetables. Don't forget to add good olive oil too, as this will allow your body to better absorb nutrients that are provided in the vegetables. Shred carrots to release the vitamin A. Table salt is pure sodium chloride and is to be avoided as it is associated with raised blood pressure and has few benefits other than taste. Sea or rock salt and mixed pepper not only provided added flavour but also give you those little extras that your body needs to maintain equilibrium. A good salt will contain a range of minerals including magnesium, which is often low in those with chronic inflammation. For this reason, always put a shake of S&P on your ferments. Another easy win to add to your vegetables is lemon or lime juice. The North Africans almost always add a splash of lime or lemon to their salads or throw in a quarter of one into the salad itself. Citrus fruit have myriad health benefits (15). Remembering to add that little bit everyday will go a long way to helping you to maintain equilibrium. I have a webinar on my website www.doctorese.com that is dedicated to showing you the benefits of salad dressing. People have even tried to patent the contents of salad dressing as a health food!

HOW DO WE REINTRODUCE OLD FRIENDS?

Start with the great base you already have established. I often start with foods that are easy to combine with the Phase II base, i.e. foods that can be fermented. This is because the fermentation process will in many cases break down mycotoxins or pesticides. Studies also show that lactic acid bacteria may even break down plastics and bind heavy metals. This means that if we ferment these culprit foods, our body may be able to cope with them without causing harm to the DNA or gut.

In Phase III, rather than introduce one individual food at a time, you may now introduce one food *group* at a time. The groups are given below.

- Fruit
- Chocolate
- Beans, hummus, lentils and seeds
- Coffee
- Breads
- Alcohol
- Milk

In Phase I and II, I described the 'wavy' reactions that you might experience during the elimination phase of Diet to Detox (Phase I) or during the fermentation phase of Diet to Detox (Phase II). I'd like to add another possible explanation for the 'wavy' reactions that you might experience during Phase III Diet to Detox. When we reintroduce old friends, we are potentially reintroducing toxins. Hence, the 'wavy' reaction in Phase III may be a toxin reaction. You'll remember that the toxins may cause direct damage to the DNA, to the gut and to our cells. These reactions can vary from being immediate to taking a few hours of days to manifest. If you should feel unwell, it is always a good idea to think back to what you ate over the preceding 24-48 hours. Immediate common reactions might be fatigue, abdominal pain and heart burn. Over the next few hours and days reactions might include diarrhoea, brain fog, poor sleep, anxiety, depression, irritability, joint pain, rash, itching, constipation, shortness of breath or a return of old symptoms.

You will note a big overlap between the different types of wavy reactions which is why I lump them all together. It can be very difficult to distinguish between a reaction that has occurred because of a 'die off' and a reaction that has occurred because of toxin damage, toxin release, biofilm breakdown or 'good' microbes ending up on the wrong side of the gut barrier. But in practice, it doesn't really matter, because either way, what the reaction tells us is that your body is in a state of dis-equilibrium.

If you experience a wavy reaction, follow the same procedure

MILD/MILD REACTIONS

If both duration and severity are mild, wait until the symptoms have calmed down and re-try the food for a further week. If the symptoms no longer return, you are free to continue eating this food. If the symptoms return, remove this food from your 'can eat list' and retry it at a later date, in 2+ weeks' time.

MODERATE/MODERATE REACTIONS

Remove this food from your 'can eat list' and re-try after 6+ weeks. If when you try it you again have a reaction, either wait another three months or generally avoid it.

SEVERE/SEVERE REACTION.

Remove this food from the 'can eat list' and re-try a very tiny portion, such as half a teaspoon, in three months or more's time. If you again have a reaction, either wait another three months or generally avoid it.

as in Phase II:

FRUIT

Fruit is a good 'old friend' to reintroduce as it is easy to ferment. Simply throw some fruit into your fermented coconut yoghurt and you'll have created a wonderful dessert or breakfast. For a simple breakfast, add the fruit to the coconut yoghurt the night before and there it is, ready for you in the morning. Or you could add ripe mango to the coconut ferment to make a creamy mousse. Of course, you don't need to use coconut yoghurt. Fruit coulis is just kombucha and puréed fruit left to ferment for 4-8 hours. You can do the same with any fruit. Just make sure that the final product doesn't taste too sweet – it should taste tart. You know that the fruit is fermenting because you'll see bubbles forming. On the rare occasion that you don't see any bubbles, sadly it is because the fruit is likely to have been sprayed with pesticides or maybe is 'dead' because it has been kept in some state of suspended animation before it is delivered to the supermarket shelves. This phenomenon is not uncommon.

You can even make fruit condiments for meat dishes or to go with fermented cabbage, such as fermented marmalade. This scrumptious Phase III fruit ferment can be added to duck or mixed with fermented cabbage to really bring you into the gourmet home cooking arena. Or how about sorbet? Simply ferment fruit with kombucha and freeze it. You can also make kombucha ice lollies this way.

CHOCOLATE

When we start fermenting chocolate we enter a whole new realm of fermented delights. To make a quick and easy chocolate ferment, take a bar of organic dark 100 % chocolate with little or no sugar. Melt the chocolate, add 2-3 dessert spoons of blackstrap molasses and some ferment (either ½ teaspoon of Ferment Blend, ½ teaspoon of kombucha or ½ tsp of coconut yoghurt). Place this in a dish that has been lined with a baking sheet and allow to set in the fridge. You can then enjoy little bits as and when you like – if you can hold yourself back. The chocolate continues to ferment as the days go by, becoming richer and richer, with hints of alcohol. If you use kombucha for the ferment, you get a spongier result.

Another favourite of mine is fermented chocolate mousse. This too is a relatively simple recipe that doesn't really go off. In the early days of my journey, I would regularly have a few dessert spoons of fermented chocolate mousse with my morning coffee. You can also make chocolate ice cream and, if you choose the sake lees ferment I mentioned in chapter 7, you will find it's particularly rich and velvety.

BEANS, LENTILS, HUMMUS AND SEEDS

The reason we leave beans, lentils and seeds until later on in Phase III is because of the anti-nutrients in the tough outer shells. This means that, quite apart from the fact that they may be culprit, toxin-containing foods, the body may find it hard to digest them in the first place. Fermentation certainly helps this process, as does grinding and cooking. Even frying can be helpful to break down some of the anti-nutrients. There are many fermented recipes in the recipe section that contain the ingredients in this group. Fermented hummus is made from chickpeas and maybe a dash of lemon, plus a ferment such as shiokoji, kombucha, kefir or Ferment Blend. For beans and lentils, soaking overnight and adding in one of these ferments can help the breakdown of culprit toxins as well as anti-nutrients. Play around with the different ferments to see which you prefer. Even after you have cooked your final dish, you can also add a ferment to allow the dish to produce even more wonderful bioactive substances. I sometimes do this with a stew that won't fit in the fridge – I simply splash in some old kombucha and leave the covered stew on the countertop.

COFFEE

Ah! Coffee! What a relief! So many people love their coffee, myself included, and it is quite possibly one of the most difficult things to give up in Phase I Diet to Detox. It's therefore one of the most pleasurable items to reintroduce. But I'd like to sound a note of caution when reintroducing this old friend, as it is one of the foods that may cause a 'wavy' reaction due to the toxins released from the coffee. For this reason, try to find mycotoxin- and pesticide-free coffee.

Even if you do find toxin-free varieties, you may still have a 'wavy' reaction when you reintroduce coffee. You might find that one cup is OK but two is not. You can kill off some of the toxins by using UV light irradiation (explained below) on your coffee beans or coffee powder before using them or mixing your coffee powder with some of my Ferment Blend. Use approximately 1 teaspoon of Ferment Blend per 500g of coffee powder and stir well. I'm not entirely sure why this works but it does seem to reduce 'wavy' reactions.

BREAD

Back in the days before I realised that my family were gluten and milk intolerant, I would make huge loaves of bread in my bread maker. There is nothing quite like the smell of fresh bread wafting through the house. Once I realised that gluten was a problem, I went through a phase of perfecting gluten-free bread in the bread maker. (The trick is to add enough eggs to make the mixture rise – I was quite proud of these offerings.) However, Luke would still get unwell with these, and we know now that this was because of the toxins. To prevent a 'wavy' reaction in Phase III Diet to Detox, think about how you're going to deal with the toxins in the flour. For example, you could pre-ferment the flour or UV irradiate it or both. The lactic acid bacteria and yeasts that work in the pre-fermentation process will help to break down plastics, pesticides and moulds and will help to bind heavy metals. UV irradiation will help to break down mycotoxins and any other microbes. Here, pre-fermentation is just the same as making a sourdough bread except that you will use gluten-free dough. You'll find some simple bread recipes in the recipe section. They are in fact a cross between a bread and a cake as you never quite get the same consistency when you use gluten-free flour, but they are just as delicious. Making a kombucha bread is as simple as mixing kombucha with gluten-free flour, leaving it to ferment for 4-8 hours, then baking it in a moderate oven until it pulls away from the side of the tin.

I tend to leave the reintroduction of gluten (and milk) to right at the end of Diet to Detox. Some people may not be able to manage regular gluten and/or milk at all. Studies show that some Africans and Asians lose the ability to digest milk with age, so do bear this in mind. I can manage to eat both gluten and milk, but not every day, or I start to get eczema and my bowels go a little 'wavy', so I tend to save my gluten and milk eating for when we go out to a restaurant.

ALCOHOL

As we learnt in chapter 6, alcohol drunk in moderation is a good thing. However, it went on the culprit list due to the presence of mycotoxins and pesticides in most beer and wine. So what do we do when we reintroduce this old friend? You can't pre-ferment it or UV irradiate it, so what to do? Well, you must choose your beer or wine carefully. Choose organic if possible but also know that, for the reasons described previously, these may still give you 'wavy' symptoms. As per coffee, you might be able to manage one glass of wine but not two. The same applies to beers and spirits.

MILK

It makes me sad to think that so many people are intolerant to milk and milk products. Real non-pasteurised, non-homogenised milk from a healthy cow that has been fed grass and not grain is full of good nutrients and wonderful bioactive substances. However, heat-treated, whizzed up milk from a cow that has been fed grain, which itself may have been subject to mould and sprayed with pesticides, is not healthy for a human to drink. Try to make wise choices when you reintroduce this old friend. You may have a local farmer who offers full-fat milk from grass-fed cows and can vouch for good animal welfare techniques. A happy, healthy animal produces happy, healthy milk. Drinking raw milk from a certified healthy animal will provide a broad spectrum of health benefits compared to drinking heat-treated (pasteurised) milk. You can find a wealth of information about the importance of making wise choices when it comes to drinking milk on the Real Milk website, set up by the Weston A. Price Foundation (16).

I am a great fan of real milk. However, I have found that

some people struggle to reintroduce this old friend completely to their life. As mentioned above, this may relate to ethnicity, or it may relate to difficulties sourcing real milk. Supermarket milk may not make the cut! For this reason, none of the recipes in the Diet to Detox recipe section contain milk. If you can source real milk, however, and you tolerate it well, feel free to substitute coconut milk for real milk.

WHAT HAPPENS AFTER PHASE III DIET TO DETOX?

By the end of Phase III Diet to Detox you should have no symptoms and be eating a varied diet of pre-fermented and raw fermented foods, fermented desserts and fermented drinks. You should also be wowing your friends and family with the *umami* of your foods. Most importantly, you should understand why you got sick and how you recovered your wellbeing.

Is the road from here on in a smooth one? Unlikely! I'm always tempted to say that there is a Phase IV of Diet to Detox. This is kind of an intermediate phase that takes you towards long-term health. Understanding Phase IV requires a trip back to the biofilm layers I mentioned in Phase I.

With my patients, I often find that the journey to wellbeing goes a little like this. We work methodically and patiently through all the phases and accept the 'waves of recovery'. We take information from each 'wavy' reaction and this helps us to understand our reaction to foods, toxins and our environment. For example, if the patient feels particularly irritable, moody or anxious, amongst other things, I understand that this might be related to something they ate. We may then want to look back at this particular food and analyse how they might modify the way they eat it. This is all important information. But I find that even once the patient is well and has no symptoms and is enjoying preparing, cooking and eating delicious new and health-giving foods, the story doesn't end there.

I notice that after a variable period of time, symptoms old or new may appear. The only adequate explanation I have for the appearance of these symptoms are biofilms. Sometimes patients might develop hay-fever symptoms they used to get as a child, or develop a urinary tract infection like they used to suffer from when they were younger. I put these 'old' symptoms down to the uncovering of a biofilm layer. Remember that I said that the characteristic of a biofilm depends on its specific environment at the time that it was formed. For example, if I use mint tea to make a batch of kombucha, the biofilms that are formed during this batch will contain mint and any products related to the breakdown of the mint by the microbes. Biofilms can be formed almost anywhere in the body, but there is still some debate about whether a biofilm is a normal phenomenon. For example, it is accepted that there are biofilms that form around the teeth. In healthy teeth the microbes are 'good' and do not cause tooth decay, but when there is tooth decay, the biofilm contains pathogenic microbes. In other places such as the lungs, gut, skin and urinary tract, it seems that small colonies of microbes are OK but larger colonies that form biofilms may be detrimental.

Biofilms are known to the medical profession because they form stubborn coatings on catheters, stents and implants, which are resistant to antibiotics and can therefore lead to chronic infection. They can be responsible for methicillin-resistant *staphylococcus aureus* (MRSA) in hospitals and nursing homes. In fact it is said that 60% of all hospital or healthcare infections are due to biofilms (17). Many probiotic foods and their wonderful bioactive substances are biofilm breakers. Lactic acid bacteria and foods such as turmeric, garlic, rhubarb and red peppers to name a few will naturally help to digest abnormal biofilms (18). As these biofilms are tough, it can take some time for them to completely breakdown. When they do, they may come away without consequence and with no associated symptoms. On the other hand, they may slough off, and patients often tell of slimy mucous in their stools associated with the return of old symptoms or the appearance of new ones.

If you can imagine that the biofilms have been building up in their various locations since birth, you can also imagine that as they breakdown and slough off, you will be removing a part of your biological history. My take on this is that the microbes that were around at a particular period in your history would have been specific to your environment at that time. If you were inhaling cigar fumes from a smoking parent, for example, the microbes would be adapted to 'eat' (or fix) cigar fumes, so the biofilm formed at this period of time would contain cigar smoke-fixing microbes and their metabolites. If you swam in a lake that was contaminated with petrol during a certain time in your life and you developed a biofilm on your head, when and if you remove sufficient biofilms layers to get to that period of your history, you might even smell petrol fumes as the biofilm layer is coming away.

Let me take this one step further. Researchers working on the quantum aspects of water, including our body water, have shown that an 'imprint' or energetic signature of our memory is stored in our body water. What if it is stored also in these biofilm layers, which after all are made up primarily of water held in the gel-like biofilm matrix? When we remove a biofilm layer we also 'uncover' memories from that period of time. This is not so far-fetched – I see many emotions accompanying biofilm removal that would support this association. For example, a patient might be doing well but then might suddenly develop a urinary tract infection that they used to get as a child. Emotions from the same period of time might also arise and need to be dealt with gently. These fascinating phenomena often occur in this unofficial Phase IV of Diet to Detox when the patient is more or less well but then gets these seemingly odd blips in their recovery.

Another phenomenon that can accompany any phase of Diet to Detox, particularly in women, is bloating and water retention. Especially in the early stages, a certain food might trigger gas production in the upper intestine, often suggesting that the patient has SIBO. The gas production can be quite dramatic and the patient will often tell me that soon after eating certain foods they look as though they are six months pregnant. This reaction will typically settle down as we get rid of the microbes growing in the wrong place in the upper gut.

Another tummy phenomenon is water retention, where the tummy may noticeably develop a pouch of fat. This can be related to eating certain foods but usually doesn't occur as rapidly as the gas-associated bloating. I believe that this is related to local inflammation in the abdominal tissues and could be due to toxin storage in this area. As I've mentioned previously, toxins are stored in various organs and soft tissues around the body. When we begin to eat the right way, including health-giving fermented foods, our body may be signalled to start to remove the toxins from their storage places. I believe that en route to being excreted they become stored in the abdominal fat, which is why I sometimes see fat pouches appearing in Phase IV. The fat pouches resolve as the body continues to deal with its toxic load.

DETOXIFICATION EQUIPMENT

A whole book could be written about detoxification equipment. This includes saunas, near and far infra-red saunas, electro-magnetic devices, cold therapy, foot spas and the like, which can be of assistance for the detoxification process. I have used many of these tools to good effect.

The equipment often helps to dislodge or remove toxins from

their storage spaces, forcing the body to eliminate the toxin. The toxin may travel out in the sweat, the blood or the lymphatics to the liver and gut or out through the kidneys and urine. The machines do a great job of releasing toxins but the body must still get the toxin out of the body, and this is where the gut plays a big role. The gut and gut microbes must transform the toxin into a format that the body can easily excrete. If you still have gut dysbiosis, this biotransformation cannot take place and the toxin circulates in the blood stream and finds another hiding place. Not only this, but the released toxin activates the Ninja peas and inflammation so that you feel rotten – and all for nothing. It is for this reason that I recommend the use of the detox machines after Phase III Diet to Detox and not before. I have also found that, when you have working detoxification pathways like those described above, you need minimal help from the machines. As soon as the body feels even vaguely back in shape, it will start to do the detoxification process itself.

This means that the machines may not be necessary. What does help, however, is exercise that promotes sweating but, as mentioned previously, only within your own safe parameters. Exercise should leave you just mildly out of breath and with very light perspiration. Exhaustive exercise will harm the gut microbes and may set you back a number of weeks. Do remember to drink good water after exercising and drink until you need to pass urine.

Another activity that helps with both detoxification and physical wellbeing is cold immersion. I used to live by the sea in Brighton, and at the crack of dawn all year round you would find a hardy group of swimmers embracing the cold water without wet suits. I find that a cold dip invigorates like very little else! Cold immersion has also been shown to reduce inflammation. But start gently. I normally suggest that my patients start with a tepid shower at the end of their normal hot shower. They should then gradually push the tap towards cold until they are having a cold shower at the end of their hot shower. Once they can manage this for three minutes, they are ready for cold immersion. If you don't have a cold sea near you, there's always a cold bath. I know this may not be so appealing but cold therapy is an easy way to both feel great and to reduce inflammation. Give it a try!

UV LIGHT

UV light has been shown to break down mycotoxins in grains. I bought a UV light bulb and have it in my kitchen. I put grains, pulses, coffee and anything that I think may be subject to mycotoxins under it. I leave them there, agitating them from time to time, for anything between four and twenty-four hours.

UV light will also create vitamin D2 in your mushrooms. Place them gill side up and leave them there for a few hours. Even if you then decide to dry the mushrooms, they still retain some of their vitamin D.

SUGGESTED FOOD COMBINATIONS FOR MEALS FOR PHASE III DIET TO DETOX

BREAKFASTS

Fermented yoghurt with fermented fruit coulis
Pre-fermented sausages or bacon with eggs and pre-fermented mushrooms
A handsome side of fermented vegetables e.g. cabbage, red peppers, olives
A side of fermented protein such as salmon, trout or hummous.
Fermented chocolate mousse
Mycotoxin and pesticide free coffee with added Ferment Blend
Kombucha, kefir
Good water

LUNCHES AND DINNERS

STARTERS
See meal combinations as per Phase II.

MAIN COURSES
See meal combinations as per Phase II.

Pre-fermented smoky beans can be made with a tomato base. The smokiness comes by adding smoked paprika. Or you could go for a totally different taste by combining the beans with coconut milk and some Chinese five spice.

A quick fermented bread goes nicely with lunch. Simply add kombucha to some pre-fermented flour – you can flavour the bread with herbs or add chunks of bacon if you like.

DESSERTS

See meal combinations as per Phase II.

Yoghurts and chocolate mousse can be made in advance and left in the fridge to mature as the week progresses. You can also make yourself some fermented chocolate and have small pieces for dessert or indeed for breakfast.

Create an easy scone like the bread in the main course. Add more brown sugarcane sugar or add fruit such as raisins or cooked rhubarb.

You'll find some delicious cakes in the recipe section, all using easy fermentation techniques.

1. Talon R, Leroy S. FERMENTED FOODS Fermented meat products and the role of starter cultures. 2014
2. Romeo J, Diaz L, Gonzalez-Gross M, Wärnberg J, Marcos A. Contribution to the intake of macro and micro nutrients exerted by moderate beer consumption. Nutricion hospitalaria. 2006;21:84-91.
3. Arranz S, Chiva-Blanch G, Valderas-Martínez P, Medina-Remón A, Lamuela-Raventós RM, Estruch R. Wine, beer, alcohol and polyphenols on cardiovascular disease and cancer. Nutrients. 2012;4:759-781.
4. Feinberg LS, Stephan RB, Fogarty KP, Voortman L, Tiller WA, Cassiani-Ingoni R. Resolution of cavitational osteonecrosis through NeuroModulation Technique, a novel form of intention-based therapy: a clinical case study. The Journal of Alternative and Complementary Medicine. 2009;15:25-33.
5. Campbell DLM, Dyall TR, Downing JA, Cohen-Barnhouse AM, Lee C. Rearing enrichments affected ranging behavior in free-range laying hens. Frontiers in Veterinary Science. 2020;7
6. Bray HJ, Ankeny RA. Happy chickens lay tastier eggs: motivations for buying free-range eggs in Australia. Anthrozoös. 2017;30:213-226.
7. Donnelly PJ, Stewart RK, Ali SL et al. Biotransformation of aflatoxin B1 in human lung. Carcinogenesis. 1996;17:2487-2494.
8. Smith GBJ, Bend JR, Bedard LL, Reid KR, Petsikas D, Massey TE. Biotransformation of 4-(methylnitrosamino)-1-(3-pyridyl)-1-butanone (NNK) in peripheral human lung microsomes. Drug metabolism and disposition. 2003;31:1134-1141.
9. Zrelli S, Amairia S, Zrelli M. Respiratory Syndrome Coronavirus2 response: Micorobiots as Lactobacilli could make the difference. Journal of medical virology. 2020
10. Fonseca S, Rivas I, Romaguera D, Quijal... M. Association between consumption of fermented vegetables and COVID-19 mortality at a country level in Europe. MedRxiv. 2020
11. Dofferhoff ASM, Piscaer I, Schurgers LJ, Walk... J. Reduced vitamin K status as a potentially modifiable prognostic risk factor in COVID-19. preprintsorg. 2020
12. Jong AY, Stins MF, Huang SH, Chen... SHM. Traversal of Candida albicans across human blood-brain barrier in vitro. Infection and 2001
13. Konecny P, Drummond FM, Tish KN, Tapsall JW. Saccharomyces cerevisiae oesophagitis in an HIV-infected patient. International journal of STD & AIDS. 1999;10:821.
14. Enache-Angoulvant A, Hennequin C. Invasive Saccharomyces infection: a comprehensive review. Clinical Infectious Diseases. 2005;41:1559-1568.
15. Mohanapriya M, Ramaswamy L, Rajendran R. Health and medicinal properties of lemon (Citrus limonum). International Journal of Ayurvedic and Herbal Medicine. 2013;3:1095-1100.
16. Foundation WAP. A campaign for real milk. Available from: https://www.realmilk.com/
17. Penesyan A, Paulsen IT, Gillings MR, Kjelleberg S, Manefield MJ. Secondary Effects of Antibiotics on Microbial Biofilms. Frontiers in Microbiology. 2020;11:2109.
18. Mishra R, Panda AK, De Mandal S, Shakeel M, Bisht SS, Khan J. Natural anti-biofilm agents: Strategies to control biofilm-forming pathogens. Frontiers in Microbiology. 2020;11

PHASE I RECIPES

PRE-FERMENTATION
In Phase I Diet to Detox you will eliminate the 'culprit' foods. The recipes in Phase I will give you some ideas about what to eat. As mentioned earlier, active live ferment is not added at this stage as it may cause a 'wavey' reaction. However, I haven't eliminated all ferments from Phase I. In particular, you will see me use the term 'pre-fermentation'.

In this situation, for the most part, the microbes will be destroyed during cooking. However, the fermentation before cooking will break down anti-nutrients such as oxalates or phytates, and toxins. At the same time the microbes will produce wonderful bioactive substances such as vitamins, peptides and anti-inflammatory/anti-oxidant molecules. The overall effect is to produce a more nutrient-dense and flavourful food.

Research suggests that whilst most of the microbes are destroyed with cooking, some do survive. This is a good thing. However, if you are new to Diet to Detox, you may want to leave the pre-fermentation recipes to the end of Phase I or even Phase II or leave out the Shiokoji and use olive oil and fresh herbs instead.

Herbs and spices

You will see that I have also used some spices in Phase I. Fresh herbs and spices that you have grown yourself are allowed as these are not likely to be subject to moulds and hopefully you will not have sprayed them with pesticides. If you are using shop bought herbs and spices, which is most people, omit these in Phase I.

SCOTCH BONNET OIL

A Scotch Bonnet is a type of hot pepper. West Africans use this type of pepper a lot in their cooking. Here I've made it into an infused oil which you can use to add fire to your soups, sauces and stews or use it as a 'shot' to give yourself a boost. The oil is rich and strong so be careful – it is fiery hot. You can keep topping up the oil as you decant it off to use it. Just make sure that all of the pepper is beneath the surface of the oil, otherwise it will come in contact with the air and go mouldy. If you don't have Scotch Bonnet, try another type of pepper.

INGREDIENTS
A handful of scotch bonnet chillies
Olive oil from a can

METHOD
Blanch the scotch bonnets in boiling hot water for 1 minute (to kill off any nasties). Drain and leave to cool down.

Once cool, add them to your fermentation vessel. Pour in enough olive oil to fill the vessel. Replace the lid, label the side with the date and leave to infuse for at least a week before using.

GARLIC OIL

This infused oil will be a wonderful addition to your kitchen. Don't peel the garlic skin off before blanching as all the good stuff is in the skin. You can keep topping up the oil as you use it. Be sure to make sure all of the garlic bulbs are beneath the surface of the oil as the bulbs in touch with the air may go mouldy.

The quantities depend on your infusion vessel rather than the proportions of garlic to oil. The more oil, the less strong the oil. Also, the longer you leave it to infuse, the stronger the oil. There is no time limit to how long you can leave this to infuse. You can start using it straight away but it will be quite weak. You'll start to notice a garlicky taste after about a week and it will become stronger after that. Once decanted out into another container, again, there is no real limit to how long you can keep it. Mine doesn't last long as I use it in almost everything, hot or cold.

I use fermentation crocks to do the infusion as they are dark and keep the mixture cool. However, if you only have a glass jar, use that and keep it in a cool dark place.

INGREDIENTS
Enough garlic bulbs to create one or two layers at the bottom of your infusion vessel
Olive oil from a can

METHOD
Blanch the garlic cloves in boiling hot water for 1 minute (to kill off the nasties).

Drain off the water and leave to cool down.

Add the garlic to your infusion vessel and fill with olive oil.

Replace the cover of the vessel, label the side of the vessel with the date and leave to infuse.

BLACKSTRAP MOLASSES

Blackstrap molasses or black treacle is normally made from a sugarcane juice. In my recipe I use dehydrated sugarcane sugar. This means that on first heating, you will quickly start to get a black syrup. 500g of sugar makes around 400mls of blackstrap molasses.

INGREDIENTS
500g whole organic unrefined sugarcane sugar
250mls hot water

METHOD
Combine the water and sugarcane sugar in a heavy pan and stir over a high heat until the mixture begins to boil. Adjust the heat so that the mixture is still bubbling vigorously but not boiling over.

For the first time heating the mixture, you will need to continue the bubbling and stirring for around 15-20 minutes or until there is a change in 'texture' of the bubbles. The bubbles will go from being individual bubbles to bubbles that seem to combine and become thicker. Once this begins to happen, turn off the heat and leave the mixture to cool down (about an hour).

Once cooled down, the mixture will resemble a black syrup. Bring this syrup to the boil again. You won't need as high a heat as previously. Again, continue to 'bubble and stir' until the bubbles change texture and become thicker. Once this happens (it usually takes around 10 minutes), turn off the heat and leave to cool down for about an hour for the second time.

The cooled down mixture should now be completely solid. This is the desired state. (If the cooled down mixture is still liquid repeat step 3 and continue from there). Add the hot water to this solid mixture and turn on the heat so that it is high enough to dissolve the solid molasses and the water. 'Bubble and stir' again until the mixture looks as though it is folding over your spoon. This should take around 5 minutes. Turn off the heat and allow the mixture to cool down.

The cooled down mixture should be a thick black syrup. If the cooled down mixture is solid, repeat step 4.

BESMA'S GARLIC SOUP

My friend Besma made this soup for me when I was ill. It is truly powerful stuff. It's a good one to have when you feel you're coming down with something. If you suffer with heartburn best give this one a miss.

INGREDIENTS
9 garlic Bulbs
20g coconut oil
1 litre of boiling water or home-made meat/fish/chicken or vegetable stock
1 tsp of salt
1 tsp Herbes de Provence
100mls coconut milk or cream

METHOD
Peel all the garlic bulbs but keep the garlic cloves whole, then 'sweat' them on a low temperature (do not allow the garlic to burn) for 20 mins until cooked (they become slightly translucent when cooked).

Add 1 litre of boiling water or homemade stock of your choice then add 1 tsp of salt and simmer on a low heat for a minimum of 20 mins.

Add 1 tsp of Herbes de Provence and cook for a further 30 mins, then remove from the heat and blend in a food processor or with a stick blender until smooth and creamy.

Return to heat and add water/coconut milk/cream to give the desired consistency.

KONJAC AND SEAWEED SOUP

Konjac noodles are made from a root vegetable and are very low calorie. This is a perfect starter for all phases of D2D but especially for Phase I. If you are on Phase II or above, add Sake Lees or Miso to the soup. With Sake Lees, a small amount (1 tsp per big pot) is enough to give great umami flavour to the soup. Miso can be stirred in after you have finished boiling the other ingredients if you want to keep some of the live microbes (if not, simply add it to the soup as it is cooking).

INGREDIENTS
1 pack Konjac noodles
1 tsp dried wakame (or other) seaweed
½ tsp fresh herbs
¼ tsp salt
250mls hot water
¼ tsp Sake Lees/Miso (optional for Phase II+)

METHOD
Bring the hot water to a simmer (add Sake Lees/Miso if using) and add the dried seaweed.

Once the seaweed has expanded, add the drained Konjac noodles, the salt and the herbs.

Enjoy straight away (or if you've added Sake Lees or Miso you can leave to cook on a low, just simmering heat for 1-2 hours).

CAULIFLOWER AND SEAWEED SOUP

This is a great winter soup and wonderful for Phase I D2D. For the other Phases you can jazz up the umami by adding sake lees.

You can also pre-ferment the cauliflower before cooking by mixing in some shiokoji and leaving for 4-12 hours.

If you don't like seaweed you can switch it out for another vegetable, but I recommend you try adding a small amount as seaweed is such a nutrient-dense food. Adding just a little seaweed will ensure you don't get the seaweed taste, but you'll get some of the good nutrients.

INGREDIENTS
1 cauliflower
1 dessert spoon dried seaweed (I often use Wakame)
Salt & pepper to taste
Mixed herbs (fresh if Phase I)
½ can organic coconut milk (optional)
1 clove garlic (optional)
Coconut oil for frying
Hot water

METHOD
Crush the garlic and fry in the coconut oil until it starts to look translucent.

Add all the other ingredients, with enough hot water to just cover the cauliflower, then simmer on a low heat for 1-2 hours.

Blend in a food mixer until smooth.

PINK VEGETABLE SOUP

What to do with the fermented red cabbage that is too tart and old-looking to eat raw? Turn it into a soup! This recipe is based on the Polish kraut soups that use old cabbage in this way. As this soup is cooked after fermentation it is suitable for Phase I as there should be no microbes in the finished soup.

INGREDIENTS
1 bowl of fermented chopped red cabbage
½ white cabbage, chopped
4-8 white mushrooms
1-2 cloves of garlic
120mls organic coconut milk
About 500mls water
½ tsp bicarbonate of soda
Salt & pepper (omit pepper in Phase I) & herbs (fresh only for Phase I) to taste

METHOD
Put all ingredients except the coconut milk in a saucepan and bring to a gentle boil until all ingredients are soft.

Blend the mixture in a food blender and put back into the saucepan and bring to a simmer.

Stir in the coconut milk and simmer for 10 minutes or until well mixed.

BESMA'S SALAD

You can change this recipe up a bit by pre-fermenting the vegetables with shiokoji or kombucha.

INGREDIENTS
1 large lettuce
1 small red onion
3-4 spring onions
2 tomatoes
1 cucumber
1 tsp fresh chopped parsley
1 tsp fresh chopped coriander leaves
For the dressing:
15mls of olive oil
5mls mustard
5mls honey
5mls lemon juice
Salt

METHOD
Chop the lettuce into thin strips.

Chop the red onion and spring onion into small pieces.

Chop the tomato and cucumber into small cubes.

Add the chopped parsley and coriander leaves and mix well with the salad ingredients.

For the dressing: Combine the dressing ingredients and whisk together using a fork before stirring the dressing into the salad.

OVEN SQUASH

This is great winter food. If you don't have garlic oil or garlic infusion, use a crushed garlic clove or, if you don't do garlic at all, leave it out.

INGREDIENTS
Squash
Garlic oil
Herbs

METHOD
Preheat the oven to 150 degrees C. Place the whole squash onto an oven tray and bake for a few hours or until it is soft and squeezable.

Remove the squash from the oven, slice it in half and remove the seeds. Drizzle on the garlic oil and herbs. Increase the oven temperature to 175-180 degrees C.

Return to the oven for 30 minutes until starting to brown around the edges.

SCRUMPTIOUS SAVOY CABBAGE

Scrumptious savoy cabbage is such an easy recipe to make and great for Phase I and all other Phases of D2D. Cabbage is a divine gift to humanity in all its forms and when we cook it on a low heat the antioxidant levels rise!

If you're being extra health conscious you can prepare the cabbage with shiokoji for 4-12 hours or overnight before using it in this recipe.

You can use other types of cabbage as well but savoy cabbage has the best flavour.

For phase II and beyond you could jazz this up by adding sun-dried fermented tomatoes and/or raisins.

INGREDIENTS
1 Savoy cabbage
¼ tsp bicarbonate of soda
1 tsp coconut oil
1 clove of garlic (optional)
½ tsp mixed herbs of your choice (fresh only, if on Phase I)
Salt and pepper (omit pepper on Phase I)
50mls hot water

METHOD
Crush the garlic and gently fry in the coconut oil on a low heat.

Chop the cabbage into strips and place in the pan with the garlic before adding the hot water – this is so that the cabbage doesn't stick and burn on the bottom of the pan.

Add the salt, herbs and bicarbonate of soda, then leave to cook on a low heat (just below simmering) for 30 mins or longer (up to 14 hours). Stir regularly so the cabbage doesn't burn.

GARLIC MUSHROOMS WITH POK CHOI

Kanten powder is a Japanese seaweed powder. It is nourishing for the gut and is useful for thickening sauces and mixes. Use fresh spices only in Phase I, but in Phase II you can add dried spices. You may also want to use garlic infusion and my fermented relish in Phase II.

INGREDIENTS
2 good handfuls of mushrooms
2 pok choi
Half a garlic clove, chopped (substitute with 10mls garlic
Infusion if making in Phase II)
Coconut oil for frying
1 tsp Kanten powder (optional)
A pinch of salt
½ tsp Ras el Hanout or five spice (Phase II only)
1 tsp Dr Ese's fermented red relish (Phase II only)

METHOD
Heat the coconut oil, then chop the mushrooms into slices and fry in the oil. Add the Ras el Hanout or five spice and the Kanten powder, if using.

As the mushrooms begin to soften, chop the pok choi and add to the pan with the mushrooms, seasoning with salt.

Cook until the pok choi is tender, then top with Dr Ese's red relish if in Phase II.

MUSHROOM AND EDAMAME BEANS

INGREDIENTS
2 dessert spoons coconut oil
2 handfuls mushrooms
1 cup edamame beans
1 tsp mixed spice or five spice (Phase II only)
5-10mls Dr Ese's Fermented garlic infusion or half a crushed garlic clove
Sea or rock salt to taste

METHOD
Heat the oil in a frying pan, then slice the mushrooms and begin to fry them. Add the five spice and stir.

As the mushrooms begin to shrink, turn the heat down so that the mixture is gently sizzling and add the garlic infusion.

In a bowl, add hot water to the frozen edamame beans and leave for 5 minutes before draining the liquid and adding to the frying pan with the mushrooms.

Cover and leave for around 15 minutes on a low heat.

ROASTED PARSNIPS, CARROTS AND SWEET POTATOES

Blackstrap molasses or black treacle if you're in the UK is 'good' sugar. It acts as a prebiotic, it protects food during heating and keeps the blood insulin down. Yes, really – even though it's a sugar. Don't be afraid to add this wonderful ingredient to your foods and ferments.

INGREDIENTS
4-6 parsnips, chopped
2-3 carrots, chopped
1 medium sweet potato, chopped
20mls garlic infusion
2 tsp mixed herbs
1 dessert spoon blackstrap molasses or black treacle
Salt and pepper

METHOD
Preheat the oven to 180 degrees C.

Combine all the ingredients and mix well.

Place in a roasting dish and roast for 30-40 minutes until the sweet potatoes are soft.

KANTEN (JAPANESE AGAR AGAR) NOODLES

These Japanese noodles taste like rice noodles but, unlike rice noodles, they are pure seaweed. The Japanese take great care to produce Kanten and it is therefore more expensive than the Chinese agar agar equivalent. The beauty of Kanten noodles is that they are exceedingly nutritious and good for your gut and they also expand after you eat them, so you feel fuller for longer. They are quite bland if served alone so do spice them up with a sauce and seasonings.

INGREDIENTS
Dried Japanese Kanten noodles
Hot water

METHOD
Rehydrate the noodles by soaking them in hot water for 15-25 minutes, depending on the desired level of softness. Don't forget about them! They dissolve completely if left.

Once at the desired texture, drain off the water and add your sauce.

BURGERS

Why buy burgers when you can make them so easily? You can add different herbs and spices to this mix, just make sure they are fresh if you are in Phase I. For Phase II and III you could swap the boiled and mashed potato for flour.

INGREDIENTS
500g minced meat
1 tsp shiokoji
1 tsp mixed fresh herbs
1 egg
1 small cooked potato or sweet potato, mashed (1 dessert spoon of plain flour in Phase II)
Half a finely chopped onion
Pinch of salt (and pepper in Phase II+)

METHOD
Mix the meat and shiokoji together, cover and leave for around 4 hours.

Preheat the oven to 180 degrees C.

Add the rest of the ingredients and combine well.

Shape the mixture into burger patties, place on a greased baking sheet and bake until brown. This will take around 30 minutes depending on the thickness. Turn them after 10-15 minutes.

RECIPES USING PRE-FERMENTATION

DETOX SOUP

When you're feeling a bit under the weather, this soup will provide a highly nutrient-dense mix to help restore your wellbeing. Better still, why not make it a regular habit to have this soup 2-3 times a month to make sure your system is ready for what may come.

The mushrooms and Natto provide a great combination of ferments that is sure to boost your levels of antioxidants. If you can't get hold of Natto, you could try using a teaspoon of my Ferment Blend instead.

Don't be put off by the green colour of this soup – it tastes delicious. Be careful though, as this soup is pretty powerful, so start with a small bowl and see what that does to your bowel motions over the next six hours or so before having more. You can also freeze portions for another time.

As we are cooking the fermented vegetables, this soup is suitable for Phase I as there are unlikely to be any microbes in the final soup, but it is still a powerful food.

INGREDIENTS
1 handful mushrooms
15mls blackstrap molasses
1 carton Natto
1tsp sake lees
1 can coconut milk
1 leek, chopped
4 cloves garlic, crushed
3tsp mixed spices or Ras el Hanout
½ tsp red chilli powder

METHOD
Combine the mushrooms, molasses, garlic and natto and stir well. Cover and leave to ferment for 1-2 days, making sure to stir them each day.

Put the mixture in a large pan and add the other ingredients. Bring to the boil then lower the heat and simmer gently for 4-10 hours.

Blend the soup in a blender until smooth, then return to the stove and heat gently until warm.

Visit www.doctorese.com

SHIOKOJI MUSHROOMS

INGREDIENTS
1 handful mushrooms
5mls shiokoji
15mls olive oil
Coconut oil for frying

METHOD
Add the shiokoji and olive oil to the mushrooms and mix until the mushrooms are coated. Cover and leave for 2-8 hours before frying in coconut oil.

LARDER SHIOKOJI AND OLIVE OIL MUSHROOMS

This recipe is great for preparing mushrooms in advance, and is especially good if you manage to pick up some mushrooms that have been reduced and you can't eat them all at once. The mushrooms will keep in a dark cupboard for a few months, although you probably will eat them before they get that far.

When you need them you can use them in your cooking, fry them in coconut oil or (in Phase II only) eat them raw in salads or combined with other pickles and ferments.

INGREDIENTS
Mushrooms of any type
Shiokoji
Olive oil
Herbs & garlic (optional)

METHOD
Remove any soil from the mushrooms by rubbing with a paper towel.

Put the mushrooms in a jar, adding the herbs and a clove of garlic if using.

Squirt in 1 tsp of shiokoji per 500ml jar, then top up with olive oil so that there is no air between the jar and the jar lid.

Cover tightly with the lid and leave in a cool, dark place until you need to use them.

SWEDE, FENNEL AND SWEET POTATO BAKE

These delicious root vegetables are scrumptious, nutrient rich comfort food.

INGREDIENTS
1 bulb fennel
1 swede
1 sweet potato
1 tsp shiokoji
1 clove garlic, chopped
20-30mls olive oil
2-3 tsp mixed herbs
1-2 tsp of salt (and pepper in Phase II and III)

METHOD
Peel the swede and the sweet potato and chop into cubes. Slice the fennel into strips.

Add the shiokoji and ferment for 4-12 hours.

Preheat the oven to 140-160 degrees C. Place the vegetables and the rest of the ingredients into a roasting pan and roast for around 1.5-2 hours or until the vegetables are soft.

PUMPKIN, CAULIFLOWER AND SEAWEED SOUP

This makes a delicious creamy soup that's ideal for those cold winter days. It's pre-fermented with shiokoji then has Sake Lees and seaweed added to bring out the umami. For Phase I be sure to use fresh herbs.

INGREDIENTS
Half a pumpkin (already cooked and removed from the skin)
1 whole cauliflower, chopped into pieces
2 tsp shiokoji
1 dessert spoon dried wakame seaweed
1 can coconut cream/milk
1-2 tsp of mixed herbs
salt (and pepper in Phase II and III)
1 tsp sake lees (Phase II+)

METHOD
Place the ready cooked pumpkin pieces and chopped pieces of cauliflower in a pan and mix with the shiokoji. Leave to ferment 4-12 hours.

Add the seaweed, herbs, salt (and pepper and sake lees, if using).

Add enough water to cover the vegetables.

Bring to a boil then turn the heat down to a low simmer and cook for 2-8 hours, or until the cauliflower is soft.

Blend in a food blender and return contents to the stove.

Add the coconut milk/cream and bring to a simmer for a few minutes.

AUBERGINE AND PEA PAN BAKE

Aubergine is much under-used. Try this very simple yet delicious combination with any meat or fish.

INGREDIENTS
1 aubergine
1 tsp shiokoji
1 tsp mixed herbs
Pinch of salt (and pepper in Phase II and III)
½ cup of frozen peas
1 ½ cloves of garlic
Good oil such as grass-fed lard, goose fat or coconut oil for frying

METHOD
Chop the aubergine into cubes and marinade for 4-12 hrs in the shiokoji.

Crush the garlic and fry on a low heat with the aubergines, herbs and salt (and pepper if using) until the oil is well soaked into the aubergines.

Add the frozen peas and stir until warmed through.

PRE-FERMENTED FRIED AUBERGINES

INGREDIENTS
1 aubergine
5mls shiokoji

METHOD
Chop the aubergine into pieces and coat with the shiokoji. Leave
to ferment for 4-12 hours before frying in coconut oil.

PRE-FERMENTED CAULIFLOWER RICE

Although this recipe uses ferment, in fact we are *pre-fermenting* the vegetables before cooking them, which means that cooking will, by and large, destroy the microbes. However, the fermenting still helps to break down anti-nutrients and toxins so that the cauliflower is better digested. Also, when the microbes in the ferment enjoy the vegetable, they produce nutrients such as vitamins and anti-oxidants. All this means that the food tastes better and is better for you!

INGREDIENTS
1 whole cauliflower
½ tsp shiokoji
½ tsp mixed herbs or spices

METHOD
Grate the cauliflower and add the shiokoji, stirring to coat. Leave to ferment for 4-12 hours before adding the herbs and/or spices, then steam until soft.

SEAFOOD AND VEG MEDLEY

This really easy dish is ideal for all Phases. For Phase I you need to heat the final dish so that it is piping hot. This way you kill off most of the microbes. For Phases II and III, you do not need to turn the heat so high.

INGREDIENTS
Handful of plum tomatoes
Handful of mixed mushrooms
10mls shiokoji
Handful of frozen or fresh fish cubes
1-2 tsp mixed herbs (fresh only in Phase I)
1 clove of garlic
Some fenugreek or coriander leaves
Salt (and pepper in Phase II and III)
Coconut oil for frying

METHOD
Combine the mushrooms, tomatoes and fish with the shiokoji in a bowl.

Stir and cover and leave to ferment for 4-12 hours.

Crush the garlic and fry lightly in some coconut oil until soft, then add the rest of the ingredients and fry gently on a low to medium heat until the mushrooms are to the desired softness or until the fish is cooked.

COURGETTE, BROCCOLI AND GARLIC TRIO

Broccoli, although packed with good stuff, can be difficult to digest. It's therefore important to help pre-digest it by fermenting it with shiokoji. For Phase I you should also make sure that the finished vegetable is soft and not crunchy.

INGREDIENTS
Handful of chopped broccoli
Handful of chopped courgette
10mls shiokoji
1 clove crushed garlic
Cracked black pepper
Pinch of salt
Coconut oil for frying

METHOD
Combine the broccoli and courgette with the shiokoji and leave to ferment for 4-12 hours.

Fry the crushed garlic gently until soft, then add the rest of the ingredients, cover and leave to cook on a low to medium heat until the broccoli is soft.

PRE-FERMENTED PORK ROLL

Ever thought of marinading your joint in Kombucha before roasting it? Try this delicious recipe. Use sweet Kombucha and not vinegar as if you use tart Kombucha vinegar your meat will be tart. For Phase I be sure to use fresh herbs and spices, but these can be replaced with dried versions in Phase II and III.

INGREDIENTS
Pork roll
Sweet Kombucha to half cover the meat
1-2 dessert spoons Blackstrap Molasses
1 tsp mixed herbs
1 tsp mixed spices
1-2 dessert spoons coconut oil

METHOD
Place the pork roll in a bowl and half fill it with the kombucha.

Add the herbs, spices and blackstrap molasses, and leave to marinade for 4-12 hours, turning at the half-way point.

Preheat the oven to 190 degrees C. Drain off the liquid and place the meat in a roasting pan.

Cover with coconut oil and roast until meat juices run clear. You can calculate an approximate time based on the weight of the meat. In general, meat can be cooked in the oven for 40 minutes per kg (20 minutes per lb).

SPICY PRE-FERMENTED MEATBALLS

These meatballs are delicious and go well with the creamy tofu and mushroom sauce (Phase II). The reason we don't add the herbs to the ferment mixture is because the herbs tend to kill off the microbes.

INGREDIENTS
1 pack of minced meat (500g)
1 small onion, chopped into small pieces
1 small bell pepper, chopped into fine pieces
3tsp Chinese Five Spice
¼ tsp red chilli pepper
¼ tsp salt
4 tsp shiokoji
2 tsp mixed herbs
Coconut oil for the roasting tin

METHOD
Combine all the ingredients except the herbs in a bowl and mix thoroughly.

Leave to ferment for 4–8 hours.

Preheat the oven to 180 degrees C. Add the herbs and mix thoroughly then, using your hands, create small meat balls and place them in a greased roasting tin

Roast for 15-20 minutes until brown.

SHIOKOJI FISH

INGREDIENTS
Frozen or fresh fish portion
3-5mls shiokoji per portion

METHOD
Coat the fish with the shiokoji. If frozen leave at least 12 hours.
If fresh, leave at least 4 hours.

Cook or fry in good oil.

SALMON AND COCONUT STEW

This delicious dish is so simple to make. You can substitute the
fenugreek leaves for coriander leaves or mixed herbs (fresh only
in Phase I). In Phase I make sure you bring the stew to a boil and
then lower the heat so as not to have any microbes in the final
dish.

INGREDIENTS
4 salmon fillets
10mls shiokoji
1 can coconut milk/cream
1-2 tsp fenugreek leaves or other green herb

METHOD
Spread the shiokoji on the fish and leave to ferment for 4-12
hours.

Place the fish, herbs and coconut milk/cream in a pan and heat
gently until just simmering for 10-15 minutes.

PHASE II RECIPES

You will already be enjoying some great Phase I recipes. Now it's time add some fermented foods. In Phase II D2D remember to add foods gradually. Adding lots of fermented foods all at once can lead to a Herxheimer ('die- off') reaction. This is where the microbes in the ferment compete with the microbes in the gut (usually the upper intestine) and cause the microbes in the gut to die, leaving inflammation, bloating and pain. By adding one new food per week, this is less likely to happen.

HERBS AND SPICES

You will see that I have included herbs and spices in phase II. You'll remember that these are omitted as they may have been sprayed with pesticides or if dried and stored, may be subject to moulds. Be sure to use fresh and spices herbs if possible. If this is difficult then think of omitting the herb/spice or reserving the recipe for phase III.

KOMBUCHA

Kombucha has been drunk for centuries and contains many beneficial microbes as well as other wonderful antioxidant, anti-inflammatory properties.

Kombucha is fermented tea – usually green or black – and requires a SCOBY to begin the fermentation process. Get one from a friend or order one from a reputable supplier.

Kombucha is living and active and produces bubbles. So be careful to 'burp' your Kombucha regularly – ideally every day – to avoid any bottle explosions.

INGREDIENTS
SCOBY and old juice
2 litres of water
3-4 tea bags
150g sugar

METHOD
Boil the water and pour onto tea bags and sugar. Stir then allow to cool.

Pour into a large jar then add the SCOBY and old kombucha juice. Cover lightly to allow any air bubbles to escape.

Leave for 5-10 days, but start tasting after 4 days. When there is a hint of vinegar/acidity, pour the kombucha into bottles.

Leave out of the fridge for 1-2 days to allow bubbles to form (burping the bottles daily) then move the bottles to the fridge.

KOMBUCHA BEER

Kombucha beer isn't real beer but it may just hit the spot for those who would like to cut back on alcohol intake. As well as providing all of the live bioactive substances in Kombucha, it also provides a source of magnesium and alkalinizing bicarbonate and just a splash of quinine which may be just a little helpful for joint disorders as well as viral and parasitic infections. The ratio of kombucha to tonic water is 1 part kombucha to 4 parts tonic water, so you can make more or less according to your taste. Magnesium and bicarbonate can have a laxative effect, so again, do adjust the quantities according to your requirements.

INGREDIENTS
Epsom salts
1/2 tsp Epsom salts
1/2 tsp bicarbonate of soda
20 ml kombucha
40 ml tonic water

METHOD
Add the Epsom salts to the kombucha and stir well.

Add the tonic water and stir again.

Add the bicarbonate of soda (make sure your glass is tall enough for to accommodate the fizz) and stir until the magnesium and Epsom salts are all dissolved.

SCOTCH BONNET FERMENT

I love to use the Scotch Bonnet and Garlic ferments as tonics. I'll take a small amount of either or both if I or the family are feeling 'under the weather'. They work a treat.

Like the Scotch Bonnet oil and Garlic oil, the amounts you use for this ferment will depend on the size of your fermentation vessel. I use fermentation crocks for this purpose as they keep the ferment cool and dark, but you can use any jar. Use a cloth over the top and secure it with an elastic band. This is to allow bubbles out but no nasties in. Use sweet kombucha as this will become sour as the fermentation proceeds. As you decant off small amounts to use on a daily basis, remove the SCOBY that will form on top of the scotch bonnet and top up with more kombucha. There's no need to replace the scotch bonnet for at least six months as it will create new and great bioactive substances for you.

INGREDIENTS
Handful of Scotch Bonnet chillies (or enough to fill 2 layers of your fermentation vessel)
Sweet kombucha

METHOD
Blanch the scotch bonnets in boiling hot water for 1 minute. Drain away the water and leave the scotch bonnets to cool down.

Once cool, add the scotch bonnets to your fermentation vessel and top up with sweet kombucha.

Cover and label the vessel and leave to ferment for at least 1 week and as long as 3 months before you begin to use this.

FERMENTED GARLIC INFUSION

This infusion is a wonderful addition to your store cupboard. Add it to food as a seasoning during cooking or add it to a salad dressing. You can also take a drop when you feel as though you are coming down with a cold.

It will keep for many months and will grow its own SCOBY if you leave it very long. This might not look very pleasant but it should taste garlicky and vinegary. The longer you leave it the more vinegary it will become, so keep it in the fridge if you want to slow down the fermentation.

INGREDIENTS
1 whole bulb of garlic with skin on
Kombucha or apple cider vinegar
2 tsp honey
Pinch of saffron (optional)

METHOD
Separate the garlic cloves and blanch in boiling water for 1 minute.

Remove from boiling water and leave to cool before putting into a clean jar.

Cover with kombucha or apple cider vinegar, add the honey and saffron and stir.

Cover lightly but do not seal as you need to allow air bubbles to escape. Label it with the date.

Leave to ferment for 5 days or more.

FERMENTED TOMATO AND BEETROOT PUREE

This scrumptious purée makes a great side dish and will keep for some weeks. It will ferment quickly so if you don't like tart ferments, keep it in the fridge. The lactic acid bacteria in the ferment acts as both a bio-preservative and a provider of great nutrients. Both tomato and beetroot are rich in antioxidants, but beetroot is an oxalate-containing food. By fermenting it, you are removing the oxalates as the microbes in the ferment will eat the oxalates as fuel. The longer you leave it to ferment, the more oxalates they eat. Buy ready-to-eat beetroot or boil it yourself until soft.

INGREDIENTS
1 medium boiled beetroot
2 dessert spoons tomato purée
10mls kombucha
10mls blackstrap molasses or black treacle

METHOD
Put the boiled beetroot, tomato purée and molasses in a food mixer and blend until smooth.

Add the kombucha, cover lightly and leave to ferment for 4-24 hours.

FERMENTED BBQ SAUCE

This BBQ sauce is better than the shop bought stuff. It also combines sugar cane sugar with kombucha which means that you'll be creating a wonderful bioactive vinegar together with the other ingredients. Remember that both tamarind and blackstrap molasses help us to detoxify from harmful toxins.

As it's fermented, remember that the sweet taste will gradually become tart, so keep it in the fridge if you want it to retain some of the original sweetness.

INGREDIENTS
4 dessert spoons sugar cane sugar
80mls water
1 tsp tamarind paste
½ tsp mixed spice or Ras el Hanout
1 tsp honey
10mls kombucha
¼ tsp smoked paprika

METHOD
Add the sugar and water in a pan and bring to the boil. Stir and keep the mixture boiling as the sugar dissolves.

The bubbles will begin to come together to form a thicker mixture that almost comes away from the pan as you stir. At this point turn the heat off and let the mixture cool down.

Once cool, add the honey, paprika, tamarind paste and mixed spices to the syrup and heat gently, stirring until everything is thoroughly combined. Turn the heat off and allow the mixture to cool.

Once cool, add the kombucha and stir again until the kombucha is combined.

FERMENTED MARMALADE

This recipe is so easy and versatile. Once made, use it as straight forward marmalade on kombucha bread or use it as a marinade on meat dishes.

INGREDIENTS
1 large orange
200g whole unrefined sugar cane sugar (or brown sugar)
2 tsp Kanten powder
300mls water
5mls kombucha

METHOD
Peel the orange and keep aside about a quarter of the rind for the final marmalade.

Separate the orange segments and place these with the remaining orange peel in a pan with 200mls of water.

Bring to the boil and then lower the heat to a simmer. Allow the mixture to simmer until the orange segments are soft and lack substance (1-2 hours).

Strain to remove the orange pieces and rind (you can use them to make SCOBY juice). You are now left with the orange juice mixture.

Cut the set aside orange peel into fine strips.

Add the strips and the sugar cane sugar to the orange juice mixture and heat gently on a simmer until the rind softens a little (20-30 minutes).

Remove from the heat and leave to cool down.

Bring 100mls of water to the boil then turn of the heat and add the Kanten powder. Stir until all the Kanten powder is dissolved and leave to cool. Just as it is starting to turn to a gel, add the Kanten mix to the marmalade, stir well and leave to completely cool down.

Add the kombucha and stir again until the kombucha is thoroughly combined into the marmalade.

KOMBUCHA TOMATOES

INGREDIENTS
15-20mls kombucha
Organic tomatoes
10-15mls olive oil
1 tsp Herbes de Provence (or mixed herbs)
Salt
Black pepper

METHOD
Add the kombucha and olive oil to the tomatoes and season with the herbs, salt and pepper.

Leave for around 4 hours.

FERMENTED EGG

Fermented egg sounds all wrong, but it's delicious. Give it a try!

INGREDIENTS
1 egg
5mls shiokoji

METHOD
Boil the egg for 7 minutes then place in iced water to cool it down.

Remove the shell.

Once cool, coat the egg with shiokoji and place in a jar.

Cover and leave in the fridge for 12-24 hours.

FERMENTED BELL PEPPERS

When fermenting with kombucha you will tend to get more fizz. When fermenting with the shiokoji rice ferment you will get a milder tasting ferment for the first few days and then it becomes more tart. Once ready to eat you can either keep your peppers covered and out of the fridge which will speed up the fermentation process or keep them in the fridge which slows the fermentation process down. Either way, do give them a stir each day (if out of the fridge) and every other day or so if in the fridge. You may get a white mouldy-looking film forming on the top. This is not harmful (as long as it's white and not green or black). Just mix it into the vegetables.

INGREDIENTS
1-3 bell peppers
Ferment – either 10mls kombucha or 5mls shiokoji

METHOD
Chop or shred the peppers into small pieces or strips.

Mix with the ferment.

Place in a jar or bowl and leave to ferment for 4-24 hours.

FERMENTED WAKAME SEAWEED

Seaweed is a staple part of the diet in Okinawa, Japan, where the inhabitants are amongst the longest lived in the world.

During storage do stir the seaweed regularly e.g. every 2-5 days, or use an airlock container that prevents bad air getting in. This will keep for a long time (weeks or months) and continue to ferment. You can use it as a side dish, in soups and stews or as part of a salad.

INGREDIENTS
Dried Wakame seaweed
15mls garlic oil (or 1 crushed garlic clove and 15mls of olive oil)
5mls shiokoji

METHOD
Rehydrate the seaweed by soaking it for about 20 minutes in boiling water.

Drain the water and add the garlic oil and shiokoji and stir well.

Eat straight away or store in the cupboard.

FERMENTED SLAW

This recipe requires a lot of patience – go too quickly and you lose the mayo with no way back. The fermented cabbage will ferment the egg. This is a good thing as it will overwhelm any bad microbes in the egg. It's still an idea to keep it in the fridge once it is made, as this slows down the fermentation so that you have a lovely creamy slaw.

INGREDIENTS
Fermented Cabbage
1 egg yolk
Olive oil

METHOD
Make the mayonnaise. Add one drop of olive oil to the egg yolk and whisk for about 5 minutes or until you get a slightly thicker and creamy consistency.

Now add another drop of oil and whisk again until it becomes a little thicker – usually another 3-5 minutes.

Keep adding single drops of olive oil until the mixture sticks to the whisk. Then add 2 drops of olive oil and whisk for 2-3 minutes and repeat, then increase to 3 drops etc. The mixture should still be sticking to the whisk.

Make the slaw. Mix your homemade mayo with the fermented cabbage and leave to ferment out of the fridge for 4-8 hours.

PRE-FERMENTED FENNEL, POK CHOI AND GINGER STIR-FRY

This stir fry makes a refreshing dish. The ginger gives it a Chinese feel.

INGREDIENTS
1-2 pok choi
1 bulb fennel
Slice of grated ginger
Dash of fish sauce
2 tsp brown sugar or raw cane sugar
1 tsp shiokoji
½ tsp hot chilli pepper
1 tsp mixed herbs
Salt and pepper
Coconut oil for frying

METHOD
Chop the pok choi and fennel into slices and add the grated ginger.

Add the shiokoji, fish sauce, chilli pepper and sugar and marinate for 4-12 hours.

Stir fry the pok choi and fennel using the coconut oil to your desired crunchiness/softness, adding the herbs, salt and pepper.

SUN-DRIED FERMENTED TOMATOES

These sun-dried fermented tomatoes are truly delicious. If you make enough you can keep them in a jar of olive oil. Chances are though, they'll be gone before they make it to the jar.

INGREDIENTS
1 bowls of cherry tomatoes
15mls kombucha
1 tsp mixed herbs
Salt and pepper

METHOD
Wash and combine the tomatoes with the kombucha, herbs, salt and pepper.

Cover and leave to ferment for around 12 hours.

Drain off any excess water and place baking parchment on a baking tray.

If you live in a hot place, leave out in the sun to dehydrate. If you can't dry them in the sun, you can dehydrate them in the oven. Keeping the oven door slightly open and on a low heat (50 degrees C), place the tomatoes in the oven for 12-18 hours.

SHIOKOJI CABBAGE

This is possibly the quickest way to ferment and eat cabbage. You can eat it within 30 minutes. The pointy cabbage is the best to use as it is softer and hence the fermentation proceeds quite quickly. However, you can use any cabbage – you'd just have to leave it for a number of hours (4-8) to allow the fermentation process to really set in before eating it. You can also leave the pointy cabbage for longer before eating it. Make some and leave it overnight to have the next day. The shiokoji rice ferment really is a wonder ferment. Use the water that is left behind for the next batch or use it in your cooking. This way you get all of the wonderful bioactive substances that you can't see but are so good for the body. Enjoy!

INGREDIENTS
1 pointy cabbage
10mls shiokoji
Salt
Pepper
Mixed herbs

METHOD
Grate or shred the cabbage into fine strips.

Mix in the shiokoji until the cabbage is well coated.

Add the seasoning and mix again.

Leave for at least 30 minutes.

CREAMY FERMENTED TOFU AND MUSHROOM SAUCE

Imagine combining the wonderful healthy effects of fermented tofu with fermented mushrooms! This sauce is the stuff of five-star restaurants, plus it's so good for you. Serve with Spicy Pre-fermented Meatballs or use it cold with salads.

INGREDIENTS
1 pack of tofu
1 handful of mushrooms
10mls shiokoji
1 can coconut milk/cream
Salt

METHOD
Chop the tofu into cubes and tear the mushrooms into smaller pieces.

Combine the tofu and mushrooms with shiokoji, cover and leave to ferment for 8-24 hours

Combine the fermented tofu and mushrooms with the coconut milk and blend in a food mixer until smooth.

To use as a warm sauce, heat very gently until just simmering.

FERMENTED PEA AND MINT PUREE

This mint purée is a posh version of the British dish mushy peas. Once made you can keep this in the fridge for a number of weeks – if it lasts that long. Use it as a side garnish or as a base for soup. It is so yummy that you may just want to eat it all by itself.

INGREDIENTS
Frozen peas
10 fresh or 1 tsp dried mint leaves
15mls shiokoji

METHOD
Boil the peas until soft.

Drain off half of the water and allow to cool down.

Add the mint and shiokoji, cover and leave to ferment for 8-24 hours.

Blend to a smooth purée in a food blender.

KIMCHI

Kimchi helps with the detoxification of heavy metals, weight loss, blood sugar control, depression, atherosclerosis, reduced blood fat levels, zinc and iron absorption and the digestion of cereals and legumes.

INGREDIENTS
1 Chinese cabbage
6 tsp sea salt
3 spring onions
1 clove garlic
1 slice fresh ginger
50-100mls water
1 chilli pepper (optional)

METHOD
Chop the cabbage into bitesize chunks and rub salt into it well, then leave for 4 hours.

Wash the salt from the cabbage with running water.

Blend the spring onions, garlic, ginger and chilli (optional) with the water in a blender, then add to cabbage and rub in well (use rubber gloves). Cover lightly and leave for 2 days.

SAUERKRAUT

Cabbage is one of the most commonly eaten vegetables worldwide, which is good as it has a high vitamin C content. Cabbage is likely to have been fermented in rice wine in Korea as far back as 37 BC. This is long before James Cook used sauerkraut and citrus fruit to keep scurvy at bay. The red chilli peppers found in Kimchi were introduced in Korea in around the seventeenth century.

INGREDIENTS
1 cabbage
Sea salt/rock salt

METHOD
Grate the cabbage and put one handful at a time into a large bowl, adding up to ½ tsp of salt after each handful and pressing down with a pestle. Depending on how fresh the cabbage is, water will begin to seep out.

Cover lightly to allow air bubbles out but no moulds from the air in.

Leave out on the side for 2 days. If the water has not covered the cabbage, add more salted water (½ tsp of salt to around 100ml of water). Some people use glass or clay weights to keep the cabbage beneath the surface of the water.

Leave for around 3 weeks.

VARIATIONS
Jazz up your kraut by adding carrots, peppers, herbs and spices.

NB Make sure your utensils are clean before use – this will prevent a bad batch. At around 2–3 weeks you may see a layer of whitish material forming at the top of the cabbage. These are yeasts and are not harmful. You can either skim them off or mix them in to the cabbage.

KOMBUCHA SALAD

INGREDIENTS
1 cabbage
1-2 tomatoes (optional)
5mls kombucha
15mls olive oil
2tsp Herbes de Provence (or mixed herbs)
½ tsp salt
Black pepper

METHOD
Chop the cabbage into thin strips.

Chop the tomato into quarters.

Add the kombucha, olive oil, herbs, salt and pepper, cover and leave for 2-8 hours.

FERMENTED CUCUMBER, ONION AND RED PEPPER PICKLE

Enjoy this ferment as a delicious side dish. Leave out some of the spices or add more of your own!

If you're not going to eat all of this at once, move it to the fridge once you have made it so that it doesn't become too tart.

You can keep enjoying this dish for many days/weeks, even when it is tart. It will simply keep on fermenting like vinegar.

INGREDIENTS
1 cucumber
1 bell pepper
½ a small onion
1 tsp shiokoji
1 tsp brown sugar
½ tsp fish sauce
½ tsp mixed herbs
¼ hot chilli pepper (or fermented scotch bonnet infusion)

METHOD
Chop or slice the vegetables and mix in the other ingredients.

Leave this mixture to ferment for 4-12 hours.

MISO NATTO

This recipe comes from my friend Yasuko, who taught me how to cook delicious Japanese dishes. Mirin is a type of rice wine which may contain varying amounts of alcohol. Both the miso and mirin add flavour to this dish. Try it with tofu steak, mixed with rice or pasta, or on toast with cheese on top.

INGREDIENTS
2 cloves garlic
15g fresh ginger
500g pork/chicken/soy minced meat
2-3 packets of Natto
1 bunch spring onions
10-30g miso (white/red/koji)
100mls mirin
1-2 tsps sugar (optional)
1 tsp soy sauce
Sesame oil

METHOD
Peel away the skin and finely chop the ginger and garlic.

Heat the oil in a frying pan and add the chopped garlic and ginger together with the minced meat and fry thoroughly.

Add the miso, mirin, sugar and soy sauce and cook for 5 minutes.

Add the Natto and chopped spring onions and fry for another 3 minutes.

FERMENTED CAULIFLOWER CRUNCH

Shock horror! Deep Frying! Deep frying in good oil (solid at room temperature such as coconut oil, lard from grass fed animals, or goose fat) is not as unhealthy as you think. It locks in flavour and preserves the inside of the food to leave you with good taste and flavour.

INGREDIENTS
1 cauliflower
5cm yam (or sweet potato)
1 cup tapioca flour
1 egg
½ tsp Chinese five spice
Pinch of salt
10-20mls water
10mls kombucha

METHOD
Grate the yam, then add it to the tapioca flour, egg and water before blending together in a mixer. Add more water if too thick until you get a thick paste.

Add a pinch of salt and the kombucha or vinegar and leave to sit for 15 mins - 4 hours.

Meanwhile prepare the cauliflower.

Chop it into bite-sized chunks and rub in the Chinese 5 spice.

When the batter is ready, coat the cauliflower in the batter and deep fry until brown.

FERMENTED TROUT AND SWEET POTATO PATÉ

INGREDIENTS
1 sweet potato
1 smoked trout fillet
Ras el Hanout or mixed spice
Salt and pepper
Ferment –10mls coconut yoghurt or 5mls kombucha or
5mls shiokoji

METHOD
Combine the ferment with the smoked trout, cover and leave for
4-12 hours.

Peel and then boil the sweet potato until soft and allow to cool.

Combine the sweet potato, smoked trout, spices, salt and pepper
and blend to a smooth paste.

Leave again to ferment for 4-12 hours or enjoy straight away.

MARMALADE CHICKEN

Marmalade chicken takes a hint from Duck á l'orange and then zooms it up a notch. This chicken is so delicious that you might find yourself eating the whole lot. You'll need my Fermented Marmalade recipe, although if you haven't made some yet (please do – it's scrumptious), you can use regular marmalade instead.

INGREDIENTS
Chicken thighs
½ tsp shiokoji per chicken thigh
1 dessert spoon Fermented Marmalade per chicken thigh
Garlic oil infusion, to drizzle

METHOD
Combine the chicken with the shiokoji and the fermented marmalade and leave to marinate for 12-24 hours.

Preheat the oven to 160C. Place the chicken in a baking tray and drizzle with garlic oil infusion.

Cook for around 30 minutes or until golden. Enjoy!

VELVETY SAKE LEES ICE CREAM

INGREDIENTS
1 dessert spoon Sake Lees
½ can coconut milk
Raw organic sugar cane or coconut sugar
½ tsp vanilla essence

METHOD
Combine all the ingredients and mix to a smooth paste in a blender.

Cover and leave to ferment for 4-24 hours.

Stir again and move to the freezer for 1 hour.

Remove from the freezer and stir again before repeating step 3.

SHIOKOJI PEPPERED STEAK

Shiokoji and meat go fantastically well together. This steak is no exception. First you let the shiokoji begin to work on the meat to break down the proteins, making them easier to digest. The microbes create other 'good for you' bioactive substances and enhance the umami (flavour) of the meat. Then we go up a notch and marinade with garlic oil which brings extra notes to your palate. The chilli then gives a great bite to the meat and the molasses bring a mellow flavour. Remember the molasses also reduces the harmful heterocyclic amines that can be formed with cooked meat.

INGREDIENTS
1 steak
10mls shiokoji
10mls garlic oil or ¼ clove of garlic and olive oil
¼ tsp red chilli powder
Salt and pepper

METHOD
Squirt and spread the shiokoji over the steak. Cover and leave to ferment for around 12 hours.

Cover the steak with garlic oil and chilli powder and make sure that the steak is well coated with all the ingredients. Leave to marinate for a further 2-6 hours.

Preheat the oven to 160C. Season the steak with salt and black pepper then coat with the molasses.

Roast until cooked through.

PHASE III RECIPES

COCONUT MILK KEFIR

Originally made in leather sacs or oak barrels, different regions of the world have different names for this fermented milk drink. The Masai tribes drink 4-5 litres per day of fermented milk and it has a whole host of health-giving properties.

INGREDIENTS
1 can coconut milk
1 dessert spoon kefir grains
2 dessert spoons puréed fruit (optional)

METHOD
Prepare the kefir grains by adding water and sugar (200mls water to 30gms of sugar). Cover and leave to ferment for 1–3 days.

Keep tasting the water each day until it loses its sweetness, then add 100mls of this kefir water to one can of coconut milk.

Add puréed fruit, if using, and cover lightly to allow air bubbles to escape.

Leave for 8–24 hours depending on room temperature and desired sweetness.

QUICK KEFIR

Normal kefir is made using kefir grains but this quick method uses my ferment blend instead.

INGREDIENTS
5ml Ferment blend
1 can coconut milk
Small handful ripe fruit

METHOD
Purée the fruit in a blender before adding to the coconut milk.

Add the Ferment blend and leave for 8–24 hours depending on room temperature and desired sweetness. Once fermentation starts you will see bubbles forming in the mix.

SCOBY JUICE

What to do with leftover SCOBY? Why not make cordial or mix it with fruit pulp and rind left over from making marmalade? When you add fresh kombucha to this mix, you'll get more fermented bioactive goodness. The amazing thing about this SCOBY juice blend is that you can keep refilling it with sweet kombucha and you'll keep getting new fresh juice for many repeats. The bioactive substances are likely to change as the fruit pulp and rind ages, but variety is king when it comes to the gut. Give it a go!

INGREDIENTS
Left-over SCOBY (size doesn't matter)
Left-over fruit pulp and rind (non-waxed)
Sweet kombucha

METHOD
Blend the SCOBY and the fruit pulp in a food blender.

Add the sweet kombucha to fill the ferment container and leave to ferment for around 3-5 days.

Strain the juice to drink as cordial or use the juice and pulp to make a SCOBY cake.

NATTO AND CASHEW FERMENTED MUSHROOM SOUP

This silky mushroom soup has a deep, delicious taste and is simply packed with nutrients.

INGREDIENTS
1 cup cashew nuts
1 pack Natto
1 cup coconut milk
2 handfuls mushrooms
Salt and pepper
Coconut oil for frying

METHOD
Soak the cashew nuts and Natto in water for 12-24 hours (the longer you leave it the more tart will be the mixture).

Blend the cashew and natto in a food mixer until smooth.

Slice the mushrooms and fry in the coconut oil until soft.

Add the blended nut/natto mixture and simmer on a low heat for around 30 minutes.

FERMENTED RED RELISH

Dr Ese's Fermented Red Relish keeps giving and giving. It will continue to ferment and become more and more tart as the days progress.

Ras el Hanout is a Moroccan spice that contains about 12 difference spices. Use a mixed spice or 5 spice as an alternative.

INGREDIENTS
4-5 red cherry peppers
1 red capsicum
1 medium onion
2 tsp tomato puree
1 tsp paprika
¼ tsp red chilli powder
1 tsp honey
1 tsp Ras el Hanout (or mixed spices)
1 tsp Dr Ese's Fermented garlic infusion (or half a garlic clove, crushed)
2 tsp capers
1 tsp Herbes de Provence (or mixed herbs)
10mls kombucha vinegar

METHOD
Chop and fry the red onion in the coconut oil until it becomes soft.

Chop the cherry peppers and capsicum into small pieces and fry with the onions, tomato puree, paprika, honey, garlic infusion and Ras el Hanout until just turning soft.

Add the capers and blend in a blender until the consistency is between soft and coarse.

Leave to cool.

Add the herbs, honey and kombucha and stir all the ingredients.

Cover with a loose lid and leave overnight in or out of the fridge.

LEEK AND JAM FERMENTED SALAD

INGREDIENTS
1 leek
1 dessert spoon marmalade
½ bell pepper
½ onion
Dash of fish sauce
½ tsp red chilli pepper
Salt and pepper
Ferment – 15mls kombucha or apple cider vinegar or 10mls shiokoji

METHOD
Finely shred the leek, bell pepper and onion.

Combine the vegetables with the ferment and the rest of the seasoning and mix well.

Cover and leave to ferment for 4-12 hours.

NIAJA BEAN PATTY

Beans are good for you, but they contain anti-nutrients that your gut doesn't like. They also may contain toxins from moulds and pesticides. Pre-fermenting them with shiokoji or Kombucha helps to break down the anti-nutrients and toxins. You can use canned chickpeas if you can't get dried split blackeye peas.

INGREDIENTS
250g dried split blackeye beans
1 egg
15-30mls water
1 tsp Ras el Hanout (or mixed spice)
1 tsp salt
5mls Ferment Blend/15mls kombucha/10mls shiokoji

METHOD
Soak the beans in water overnight with the Ferment Blend, kombucha or shiokoji.

Drain the water and add the egg, Ras el Hanout and salt.

Blend in a blender to a smooth paste, adding just enough water to bring the mixture together.

Make into small round flat balls and fry in coconut oil.

GOAT AND BEAN STEW

Goat is not cooked often in the UK but is enjoyed in Africa and the Caribbean, where goat curry is a favourite dish. Its flavour is similar to but more intense than lamb. Goat meat is rich in oleic acid, the same as is found in olive oil.

INGREDIENTS
Around 2kg of goat pieces
500g passata
2 cans of ready cooked mixed beans
2 red onions
30mls red palm oil
30mls coconut oil
2 tsp Ras es Hanout or Moroccan spice
1 tsp Herbes de Provence
1 tsp sea salt
15mls Dr Ese's garlic infusion

METHOD
Chop the onions and fry in the coconut oil in a large pan before adding the rest of the ingredients.

Mix well and either cook in a pressure cooker on high pressure for 35 minutes or slow cook at 120 C for around 8 hours.

FERMENTED HUMMUS

There are a lot of different formulations for hummus. Some add tahini, but you can also mix it up by adding cooked bell peppers or exotic spices.

INGREDIENTS
1 can chickpeas
20mls kombucha
Juice from ½ a lemon
Salt and Pepper
Mixed herbs/spices

METHOD
Pre-ferment the chickpeas in their water with the kombucha for 4-24 hours.

Drain the water from the fermented chickpeas.

Blend in a mixer with the lemon juice, salt, pepper and herbs – you may need to add a little water to allow the mix to come together.

FERMENTED ORANGE SAUCE

For this, you'll need my Fermented Marmalade. This is a quick and easy orange sauce that you can use to bring tangy scrumptious flavour to meat dishes. It also tastes great poured over raw fermented vegetables.

INGREDIENTS
4 dessert spoons Fermented Marmalade
100-200mls olive oil

METHOD
Combine the Fermented Marmalade and the olive oil and warm gently in a pan until the marmalade is dissolved.

Pour over meat or any other dish.

FERMENTED RED BEAN STEW

Beans are a wonderful prebiotic food but can be harsh on the gut, particularly if you have gut dysbiosis (leaky gut). Soaking and fermenting them before cooking helps to break down some of the anti-nutrients but also provides more bioactive substances such as antioxidants. Leave out the chilli if you are not into hot things.

INGREDIENTS
1 dessert spoon shiokoji
2 dessert spoons red palm oil
2 dessert spoons coconut oil
2 cans mixed beans
1 red capsicum pepper
1 can chopped tomatoes
2 dessert spoons tomato puree
½ tsp smoked paprika
1 tsp Herbes de Provence or mixed herbs
10mls Dr Ese's Fermented garlic infusion or half a crushed garlic clove
1 tsp Ras el Hanout or mixed spice
1 tsp sea or rock salt
1 tsp honey
1 tsp red chilli powder

METHOD

If canned, pour the beans into a bowl and add the shiokoji.

Cover and leave to ferment overnight.

If not canned, soak the beans in water overnight, then soak again overnight with added shiokoji.

When the beans are ready, heat the coconut oil in a frying pan.

Coarsely chop the capsicum and add to the pan with the spices and stir.

As the capsicum begins to soften, turn the heat down so that the mixture is gently sizzling and add the garlic infusion. Stir and leave to sizzle for about 3 minutes.

Add the chopped tomatoes and blend the whole mixture in a blender until smooth.

Add the canned beans, Dr Ese's powders, tomato puree, salt, honey, Herbes de Provence, pepper and smoked paprika and stir.

Cover and leave to cook slowly for 1-6 hours, stirring every so often so the stew doesn't stick to the bottom of the pan.

ROASTED HONEY AND RAISIN FERMENTED CARROTS

Jazz up the simple carrot and turn into this luxurious dish with not too much effort.

INGREDIENTS
Handful of carrots, chopped
2 dessert spoons raisins
10mls shiokoji
1 tsp honey
1 tsp mixed herbs
Organic coconut oil, for roasting

METHOD
Place the chopped carrots, raisins, honey and shiokoji in a bowl and mix thoroughly.

Leave to ferment for 8-12 hours.

Preheat the oven to 160 degrees C. Add the herbs and roast for around 30 minutes or until the carrots are soft.

SALMON MOUSSE

Johanna Budwig recommends flaxseed oil and quark for cancer sufferers. You can add your own quark to this recipe but I find that even on Phase II some people still react to milk products so in general I don't include them in my recipes. I've substituted the quark for salmon.

Normally the omega 3 oil in flaxseeds are poorly absorbed, but in this case it combines with the sulphur amino acids in the salmon and can pass quickly into the body. You'll notice the difference in your skin almost immediately. Just be sure to incorporate all the oil into the mixture.

Some arthritis sufferers notice a difference to joint pain quickly with this formulation.

For Phase I, omit the shiokoji ferment.

INGREDIENTS
1 sheet smoked salmon
60ml cold pressed flaxseed oil
10-30ml water
½ tsp shiokoji

METHOD
Combine all ingredients and 10mls of water and blend in a freestanding mixer or with a hand whisk. If the mix is too thick add more water until you reach the desired consistency.

VARIATIONS
Use tuna instead of salmon for a cheaper option.

Use coconut milk instead of water to increase the creaminess.

LEFTOVERS PIE

This recipe uses my Fermented Pastry and is a great way to transform Sunday roast leftovers. I haven't included quantities here, but 500g of pastry will make a pie base and lid that will feed around 3-4 adults using a medium-sized baking tin. Your pie interior can be a combination of meat, fish and chicken left over from a previous meal. The important thing about the pie mix is that it shouldn't be too loose, so bear in mind that, while you need some moisture, you don't need as much as you might have in a stew. The flour and water mixture will thicken up the liquid to ensure it stays in the pie. Remember also that when you bake the pastry blind it will shrink, so make sure you create the sides of your pie slightly higher than the pie tin.

INGREDIENTS
Meat, fish or chicken leftovers
Frozen peas or leftover vegetables
GF flour and water to thicken
500g Fermented Pastry
1 egg
10mls coconut milk
Mixed herbs
Salt and pepper

METHOD
Make the pastry according to my Fermented Pastry recipe.

Preheat the oven to 180 degrees C. Take two-thirds of the pastry, roll it out and use it to line your pie tin, leaving the final third for the pie lid.

Combine the egg and coconut milk and baste the pastry base well.

Bake the pastry without the pie filling (blind) for around 25 minutes or until golden brown.

Remove from the oven and let the pie base cool slightly. You can transfer the base to a flat oven tray if preferred.

Whilst the pastry is baking, make your pie mix. Combine your leftover meat/fish and add any leftover vegetables (or frozen peas) to a pan and heat gently – just enough to melt the juices.

If the pie mix is quite loose, mix 2tsp of flour with 4tsp of water and add to the pan, stirring, to thicken the juices. Add more until you get the desired thickness – the sauce should be somewhere between runny and gel-like.

If the leftovers are quite dry, add a little water until you get the desired thickness.

Add herbs, salt and pepper and stir well, then leave the pie mix to cool slightly.

Once the mixture has cooled down, add it to the baked pie base.

Use the remaining pastry to add a pie lid, basting well with the remaining egg/coconut milk mixture.

Return to the oven and bake for approximately 30 minutes, or until the lid is golden brown.

CRISPY VEGETABLE MOUNTAIN

I just love this recipe. It is reminiscent of Onion Bhaji. I often use fermented cabbage that is too sour and mix with onions and any other veggies that I have around. I usually have some fermented flour and egg mix going in the fridge so it's easy to whip some of this out and combine it with the shredded vegetables. I have a deep fat fryer and I use good oil in it (coconut oil) and change the oil when it has gone brown. If you don't have a deep fat fryer, use a small, heavy pain and fry in small batches. The flour and egg mix (batter) gives this a delicious crispy exterior. It's great as a starter or alongside a main course and is very filling.

INGREDIENTS
1 mug plain flour
1 egg
1 small to medium cabbage, shredded
1 small or medium onion
1 carrot, shredded
½ tsp mixed herbs or spices
Salt and pepper
30mls kombucha

METHOD
Make the batter by combining the flour, egg and kombucha into a smooth, just runny paste, adding more kombucha if needed.

Leave the batter to ferment for 4-24 hours.

Combine the shredded vegetables, herbs and spices in a bowl and mix thoroughly. Season with salt and pepper.

Add the batter to the vegetables and mix thoroughly.

Heat up your good oil (test a small piece of the mixture to check that it sizzles when you add it) and add portions of the vegetable mix. Deep fry until golden, turning as necessary.

Drain off any excess oil.

SPICY FRIED CHICKEN

You can use gluten free flour instead of tapioca and almond flour.

INGREDIENTS
8 chicken wings
100mls miso paste
1 cup tapioca flour
½ cup almond flour
Ras el Hanout or Chinese 5 spice
Pinch of salt

METHOD
Marinade the chicken overnight or for a few hours in the miso paste.

Combine the tapioca flour and almond flour, spices and salt, then roll the chicken in the flour mixture.

Deep fry in coconut oil for 3-5 minutes or until deep brown.

CASHEW AND NATTO PORK BELLY

You will be rewarded for the small amount of effort it takes to make this mouth-watering dish.

INGREDIENTS
Pork belly
Handful of cashew nuts
1 pack Natto
Herbs
Salt and pepper

METHOD
Soak the cashew nuts and Natto in water for around 8 hours.

Blend into a smooth liquid.

Marinate the pork belly in the liquid for 4-8 hours, turning every few hours to ensure all of the meat gets a chance to marinate.

Add a shake of herbs and some salt and pepper.

Bake in a moderate oven until meat is cooked.

KOMBUCHA BREAD

This bread is so simple you'll wonder where it's been your whole life. It's kombucha, eggs and flour and a little of what you fancy to jazz it up. Unlike shop-bought bread or even other homemade recipes, you're using more than one fermentation micro-organism (kombucha), which means you'll be producing lots more and varied bioactive substances. You can keep a portion of this mixture in the fridge as a starter culture for when you want to make another batch. The longer you leave the mix to ferment the more bioactive substances you'll get. Although watch out – the longer you leave it the more sour the mixture becomes.

The quantities are not really that important. It is more important to understand the texture needed to produce your preferred bread. When using gluten free flour your mixture needs to be a lot softer and almost runny to give a light, moist dough. If your mixture looks too firm, add more kombucha. If your mixture looks too runny, add more flour. It's as simple as that. You also don't need to knead gluten free flour.

INGREDIENTS
3 mugs gluten free self raising flour
2 eggs
2 mugs kombucha
1 dessert spoon sugar cane sugar
½ tsp salt
1 tsp herbs (optional)

METHOD
Combine all the ingredients and mix until smooth.

Cover and leave to ferment for 4-12 hours.

Preheat the oven to 160C. Turn the dough into a lined or greased tin and bake for around 40 minutes or until the bread is risen and shrinks from the sides of the pan

NUTTY NATTO KOMBUCHA BREAD

The ferment in this recipe is like a sourdough starter mixture. The quantities are not critical and hence are not given. Natto usually comes in sachets or pots. To keep the ferment going, feed the dough each day with any carbohydrate- or protein-containing ingredient e.g. flour, coconut, natto, linseeds or nuts and stir. Keep the mixture in the fridge if you're not going to use it within the next 4-8 hours.

The amount of sugar you use for this bread is also up to you. The ferment will feed on sugar so it is a good idea to use at least a small amount.

The end result will vary in the way that it rises dependent on the ingredients you use. Enjoy experimenting!

INGREDIENTS
For the Nutty Natto ferment:
Nuts
Natto
Kombucha
Plain flour
Eggs
Herbs
Self raising flour
1-2 tbsp organic sugar

METHOD

Make the ferment. Combine the nuts, Natto and plain flour together, then add enough kombucha to bring the mixture together into a thick batter.

Leave overnight and then blend together in blender.

Make the bread. Preheat oven to 145°C.

Use 1 egg per portion of Nutty Natto ferment – the egg should be at least as big as the portion of Nutty Natto. Then add 1-2 more eggs depending on how much you want the mixture to rise. Whisk the eggs.

Use roughly 1 part Nutty Natto ferment to 4 parts self raising flour.

Mix the dough and flour together and fold in the sugar and the eggs.

Add the herbs and leave the mixture to sit for about 1 hour.

Grease a pan with oil and add the mixture, then bake in the oven for 45 minutes to 1 hour.

VERY BERRY YOGHURT

INGREDIENTS
10mls kombucha
1 can organic coconut milk
1 bowl fresh berries

METHOD
Add the kombucha to the berries and the coconut milk and leave to ferment for a further 4-12 hours.

FERMENTED PASTRY

Once you're well into Phase II, you'll enjoy making delicious pastries. This fermented pastry is very simple and doesn't take long to make.

I always use gluten free flour, which behaves differently to normal flour. In particular, it doesn't roll into sheets very well. Don't worry about it though – I tend to do any large pans piecemeal. I take small amounts of pastry, flatten them with my hand and put them into the greased pan, repeating until the pan is covered. I do the same with the top if making a pie. It tastes the same.

INGREDIENTS
500g gluten free flour
250g beef dripping/lard
2 egg yolks
2 dessert spoons brown sugar
10mls kombucha
Water

METHOD
Cut the lard into small pieces and rub into the flour until the mixture resembles fine breadcrumbs.

Stir in the sugar.

Add the egg yolks and kombucha and enough water to be able to bring the mixture into a ball. It is better to have the mixture slightly wetter as you can always add more flour if needs be.

Leave this to ferment for 4-12 hours.

Use as required.

SAKE LEES BATTER

INGREDIENTS
1 dessert spoon Sake Lees
4 tbsp plain flour
1 egg
100-200mls water
Pinch of salt
1 dessert spoon raw organic cane sugar

METHOD
Put all the ingredients and around 100mls of water in a blender and blend to produce the batter.

Add more water or flour to give the desired consistency – the batter should be pourable.

Leave to ferment for 4-24 hours. Stir again and add more water if needed as the mixture will thicken as it ferments.

Use as a batter by dipping vegetables or proteins in the batter and frying in good oil.

KOMBUCHA PANCAKES

You can have a pancake batter on the go all the time. Just save some from the batch you are making and add more of the ingredients and keep it in the fridge overnight or until you need it. If you're not using it the next day, be sure to give the mixture a stir and keep it covered.

INGREDIENTS
250g gluten-free plain flour
1 egg
250mls kombucha
100g raw organic cane sugar
Pinch of salt
½ tsp vanilla essence

METHOD
Combine all the ingredients together and whisk or blend until smooth.

Add more kombucha or more flour to give the desired texture for the pancake batter.

Cover and leave to ferment for 4-24 hours.

Add more kombucha to thin out the mixture as it will thicken during the fermentation process.

Take spoonfuls of the mixture and fry in hot good oil (such as coconut oil), flipping halfway through cooking.

FERMENTED VICTORIA AND BERRY SPONGE

This twist on the delicious Victoria sponge classic will be easier to digest and is just as scrumptious. What's not to love?

I use gluten free flour. Gluten free pastry and cakes need to be a little runnier than gluten containing mixes. If not they can be very hard and cardboard-like.

The longer you leave the cake to ferment the less sweet will be the final product, so play around with ferment times to see which you prefer. And yes – that means you'll have to make this more than once!

INGREDIENTS
175g gluten free self raising flour
175g organic cane sugar
175g of coconut oil
2 tsp vanilla essence
15mls kombucha

For the icing:
500g icing sugar
200g coconut oil
1 tsp vanilla essence
3 dessert spoons water
Frozen or fresh berries
Strawberry jam for the filling

METHOD
To make the cake, combine all the cake ingredients and beat until you get a soft, thick paste. Leave to ferment for 4-12 hours.

Preheat the oven to 160 degrees C. Turn the mixture into two greased and lined cake tins and bake for 30-40 minutes or until the cake has shrunk from the edges of the tin. Turn onto a wire tray to cool down.

To make the icing, combine the sugar and the coconut oil. Add enough water to make a thick, spreadable paste, adding more water if required. Defrost the berries.

Take a spatula and spread half the icing onto one of the cakes. Spread jam onto the icing and place the second cake on top.

Spread the rest of the icing on top of the cake. Decorate with the berries.

Visit www.doctorese.com

FERMENTED CHOCOLATE MOUSSE

This delicious fermented chocolate mousse can be made and left in the fridge so that you can enjoy it over about 7-10 days. As the days go by, the chocolate continues to ferment, giving a more and more intense flavour. I made some for my friend Yasuko. She managed to eek it out to 14 days.

INGREDIENTS
150g dark chocolate (70% cocoa solids)
6 eggs, separated
100ml fermented coconut yogurt (Kefir)

METHOD
Melt the chocolate in a glass bowl placed inside a pan of boiling water. Allow to cool for 4-5 minutes.

Separate the eggs and add a teaspoon of the slightly cooled melted chocolate to the egg yolks (to prevent the egg yolks from cooking) and stir.

Continue adding the chocolate to the egg yolks, stirring all the time until all the chocolate is combined with the egg yolks.

Add the fermented Coconut yoghurt and blend with the eggs and chocolate.

Whisk the egg whites until light and fluffy and forming soft peaks, then gently fold into the mixture above so you don't lose any air. This will keep the mousse light and airy.

Cover the mixture and leave out of the fridge at room temperature for around 2 hours. After 2 hours the mixture should be starting to set. Move to the fridge for 1-2 hours before eating.

FERMENTED MANGO MOUSSE

INGREDIENTS
1 *handful ripe mango pieces*
10-20mls kombucha
½ can coconut milk

METHOD
Add the kombucha to the mango pieces and stir.

Cover and leave to ferment overnight out of the fridge.

Combine the mango with the coconut milk and blend in a mixer to a smooth paste.

Leave to ferment again for 4-24 hours.

FERMENTED FRUIT COULIS

Fruit contains fruit sugar and good stuff by the way of antioxidants, but the fruit sugar is still sugar and can encourage growth of 'bad' microbes in the gut. Fruit can also be subject to mould and have been sprayed with pesticides. By fermenting the fruit, not only are you getting rid of some of the sugars but the good microbes will be dealing with some of the toxins.

If you don't have kefir or Kombucha you could use apple cider vinegar (with the mother, i.e. alive)

This recipe makes a small pot.

INGREDIENTS
1 *cup of frozen berries*
10mls fermented water kefir or kombucha

METHOD
Combine all the ingredients and leave to ferment for 1-5 days or until mixture reaches your desired tartness.

FERMENTED GLUTEN-FREE WAFFLES

This is such a simple recipe. Make it and keep some in the fridge so you can make more the next day. It will be tarter the next day and beyond so you may need to add more sugar (I prefer blackstrap molasses because of all the wonderful things it does for the gut and how it keeps insulin levels low).

INGREDIENTS
125g gluten free flour
1 egg
10-30mls fermented yoghurt or kombucha (or 1/2 tsp ferment blend)

METHOD
Combine the flour, eggs, yoghurt, and ferment (yoghurt or kombucha or ferment blend) in a bowl and mix until smooth. Add more yoghurt/kombucha or more flour as needed until you have a soft, runny paste.

Leave to sit for 15 mins–8 hours depending on how tart you like the taste.

Give the mixture another stir and add more liquid or flour if needed.

Pour batter into a waffle maker and heat until brown.

INES'S FERMENTED CHOCOLATE CHIP COOKIES

INGREDIENTS
1 cup melted coconut oil
½ cup granulated sugar
4 large eggs
½ tsp vanilla extract
300g self raising flour
1 tsp baking soda or 3-4 tsp of baking powder
Chocolate chips
½–1 tsp Ferment Blend or 5-10mls kefir or kombucha

METHOD
Whisk the oil and sugar until light in colour.

Add the eggs and vanilla extract and mix until smooth.

Add the flour, baking soda/powder, Ferment Blend/kefir/kombucha and fold until a smooth dough is formed.

Fold in the chocolate chips and leave to ferment for 2-24 hours.

Preheat oven to 375°F/190°C.

Spoon balls of the mixture onto a baking tray lined with parchment paper and bake for around 15 mins.

FERMENTED CARROT CAKE

This recipe makes a deliciously moist carrot cake. Fermenting beforehand allows the microbes in the kombucha to start to pre-digest the grains and also detoxify from pesticides and moulds. They also make new bioactive substances. Switch out the lemon icing for vanilla essence or grated carrot if you prefer not to have the lemon flavoured icing.

INGREDIENTS
100g grated carrot
150g gluten free self raising flour
100g organic cane sugar
100g coconut oil
4 eggs
40mls kombucha
For the icing:
2 dessert spoons icing sugar
Squeeze of lemon juice
¼ tsp lemon rind

METHOD
Add the grated carrot, flour, sugar, eggs and oil into a bowl and combine until smooth. It sometimes helps to melt the coconut oil beforehand.

Stir in the kombucha, cover and leave to ferment for 1-4 hours.

Preheat the oven to 160C. Pour the mixture into a greased or lined round shallow cake tin and bake for around 30 minutes, or until the sides of the cake are pulling away from the tin.

Place onto a wire rack to cool down for about 10 minutes.

To make the icing, combine the icing sugar, lemon juice and lemon rind until smooth.

Spoon the mixture onto the cake whilst it is still warm so that it will seep into the cake.

FERMENTED CHOCOLATE BITES

If you've watched my video on Good Sugars at *www.doctorese. com*, you'll know that some sugars are good for us. Here, I'm using raw, unrefined sugar cane sugar which contains wonderful bioactive antioxidants. It's combined with chocolate, which also has wonderful bioactive antioxidants, so you're getting a double whammy. I sometimes add some of my leftover coffee powder to this, as it makes it even more delicious. The ferment means that this recipe will just keep on giving if you leave it over a few days (it is unlikely to last that long). You could also jazz it up by adding a pinch of hot chilli powder.

INGREDIENTS
4 dessert spoons raw unrefined sugar cane sugar
45g chocolate (70% cocoa solids)
1 tsp leftover coffee powder (optional)
5mls kombucha
3 dessert spoons water

METHOD
Add the water and sugar to a pan and heat to dissolve the sugar, turning the heat higher until the mixture is bubbling.

As you continue to heat the mixture the bubbles will change in texture and look thicker and almost come away from the bottom of the pan as you stir. It can take a few minutes to reach this point. This will ensure that your final Chocolate Bite isn't too runny. Once at this point, turn the heat down and add the chocolate, broken into pieces, until it is dissolved. You may also add your leftover coffee powder at this point and stir thoroughly.

Allow the mixture to cool for 5-10 minutes but ensure that it is still pourable.

Line a small dish with baking parchment and pour the mixture into the dish. Leave to cool for around 20 minutes then pour the kombucha onto the top of the mixture.

Allow to harden in the fridge for a further 30 minutes before cutting into pieces.

CHOCOLATE CARAMEL SLICES

This delicious dessert almost seems forbidden it's so scrumptious. Well, it's not! It's made with wonderful sugar cane sugar which you effectively make into molasses as you use it in this recipe. Just imagine all those wonderful bioactive substances combined into something so delicious.

If you are on phase I D2D, you can make this but omit the shiokoji.

INGREDIENTS
4 dessert spoons raw unrefined sugar cane sugar
45g chocolate (70% cocoa solids)
1 tsp leftover coffee powder (optional)
5mls kombucha
3 dessert spoons water
For the caramel:
1 tsp vanilla extract
100mls coconut milk
2 dessert spoons sugar cane sugar
1 egg yolk
2 dessert spoons chopped roasted nuts

METHOD
Follow step 1 and 2 from the Fermented Chocolate Bites recipe.

Fold two-thirds of the roasted nuts into the chocolate mixture. Pour into a small dish lined with greaseproof paper. Set to one side or in the fridge to harden.

Once hardened, spoon the shiokoji onto the top of the chocolate and spread it as evenly as you can to cover all the chocolate.

To make the caramel top, add around 10mls coconut milk to the egg, stir and leave aside for later.

Add the sugar, the rest of the coconut milk and the vanilla to a pan and bring to a simmer.

Continue to simmer until the mixture is reduced by around one third of its original volume. The more reduced it becomes, the firmer the finished caramel top.

Once reduced, allow to cool for around 5 minutes before beginning to add the egg, little by little, stirring as you go. The mixture will become lumpy – this is OK – it will still taste scrumptious.

Leave the caramel mixture to cool for a further 5-10 minutes before spooning it onto the hardened chocolate. Sprinkle the rest of the roasted nuts onto of the mixture.

Place in the fridge to firm up for around 1 hour.

Once firm (the top will still be soft but shouldn't be runny), cut into slices.

FERMENTED PUFF PASTRY BALLS

INGREDIENTS
2 cups plain flour
100mls of Kombucha
5mls shiokoji
½ tsp ground nutmeg
Pinch of salt
½ cup sugar
Coconut oil, to fry

METHOD
Combine all the ingredients and mix into a thick batter.

Leave to sit for 45 minutes.

Spoon out dessert spoons of the batter into hot coconut oil, turning them over once until golden.

SCOBY CAKE

What else can you do with leftover SCOBY? Make cake! SCOBY contains some great bioactive prebiotic substances that are great for the gut. Most of the microbes might be lost during baking, but not all of them are, and it's my experience that fermented cakes and mousses keep on fermenting after they are baked. Try it and see. They don't tend to 'go off' like normal cakes. They just get better for you, at least for a few days.

INGREDIENTS
300g gluten-free self raising flour
100g coconut oil
100g SCOBY
4 eggs
100 gm sugar cane sugar
1 orange and shredded rind

METHOD
Put all the ingredients into a bowl and blend until smooth.

Cover and leave to ferment for 4-12 hours.

Preheat the oven to 150C. Pour the mixture into a greased or lined cake tin and bake for around 30 minutes or until the cake comes away from the sides of the tin.

Turn onto a wire cake rack and leave to cool.

Decorate as desired.

INDEX OF SUBJECTS

There is an Index of Recipes on page 229. Page numbers in italics indicate a figure.

immune response 28–30, 45

immunocompromised individuals 105

immunosuppressive medication 81–82

implants, as source of toxins 80

indigenous populations 34, 36

indigestion 73

inflammation

   cholesterol and 92

   chronic 19, 23, 29–30, 45–47, 67, 79–80

   as immune response 28–30, 45

   mood and 19

   omega-3 oils and 91, 191

   symptoms related to chronic 23, 32, 41–42

   toxins and 26, 49–50

Inuit populations 36

Japan 98, 99–100

Jarisch–Herxheimer (die-off) reaction 82

joint problems

   calcium oxalate deposits 88

   kombucha beer and 154

   mould toxins (mycotoxins) as cause of 14, 54

   omega-3 oils and 91, 191

   osteoarthritis 17–18, 19, 79–80

juicing 88–89

Kanten noodles 137

Kanten powder 134

kefir 100

kefir water 103

ketones 35–36

kidney function 93

INDEX OF RECIPES

CPSIA information can be obtained
at www.ICGtesting.com
Printed in the USA
LVHW112041210322
713998LV00014B/1291